FIELD MANUAL
No. 21-11

HEADQUARTERS
DEPARTMENT OF THE ARMY
WASHINGTON, D.C., *28 May 1970*

FIRST AID FOR SOLDIERS

			Paragraph	Page
CHAPTER	1.	GENERAL	1–6	3
	2.	LIFESAVING MEASURES A B C D		
Section	I.	Lifesaving Measures A: Clear the *Airway* and Restore Breathing and Heartbeat as Necessary	7–9	10
	II.	Lifesaving Measures B: Stop the *Bleeding*	10–12	24
	III.	Lifesaving Measures C: Administer Shock *Control*	13, 14	31
	IV.	Lifesaving Measures D: Apply *Dressing* and Bandage	15–19	33
CHAPTER	3.	INJURIES REQUIRING SPECIAL FIRST-AID MEASURES		
Section	I.	Severe Wounds and Burns	20–25	67
	II.	Fractures	26–32	73
CHAPTER	4.	COMMON EMERGENCIES	33–45	92
	5.	TRANSPORTATION OF SICK AND INJURED	46–48	103
	6.	FIRST AID IN A TOXIC ENVIRONMENT	49–60	125
	7.	PSYCHOLOGICAL FIRST AID	61–66	140
APPENDIX	A.	REFERENCES		149
	B.	CONTENTS OF FIRST AID CASE, KITS, AND PACKS		150
INDEX				153

***This manual supersedes FM 21-11, 22 July 1959 including all changes; and paragraphs 8-31, 33-37, 39-42, 45-51, 56, 57, 61-66, 69-76, and 92-96 of FM 8-50, 6 June 1957, includng C 1, August 1965.**

CHAPTER 1
GENERAL

1. Purpose and Scope

The purpose of this manual is to help you understand the importance of first aid to an injured person and to provide you with an explanation of the first aid measures which you can apply to yourself and to other persons before trained medical personnel arrive. This manual contains instructions in lifesaving measures, including how to clear the upper airway, to give artificial respiration and closed-chest heart massage, to stop bleeding, to control shock, and to protect the wound. It describes special measures which you should apply for specific kinds of injuries, common emergencies, and injuries resulting from contact with toxic substances. It also explains improvised methods of transporting the sick and injured and presents some basic principles and methods of psychological first aid. Publications to which references are made in this manual are listed in appendix A. The contents of the first aid case, kits, and packs are listed in appendix B. Also, the first-aid provisions of STANAG, CENTO STANAG, and SEASTAG No. 2122 have been implemented in this manual.

2. Maintenance of Manual

Users of this publication are encouraged to submit recommended changes to improve the publication. Comments should be keyed to the specific page, paragraph, and line of the text in which the change is recommended. Reasons will be provided for each comment to insure understanding and complete evaluation. Comments should be prepared using DA Form 2028 (Recommended Changes to Publications) and forwarded direct to the Commandant, US Army Medical Field Service School, Brooke Army Medical Center, Fort Sam Houston, Texas 78234.

3. Importance of First Aid

a. First aid is the care given to casualties before treatment can be administered by medical personnel. The Army Medical Department has the finest equipment available, and its personnel have been trained in the most modern methods of saving life and easing pain. Medical personnel, however, cannot be everywhere at once; there may be a time when YOU will have to depend upon your knowledge to save YOUR OWN LIFE or the LIFE OF SOMEONE else. You may be able to save a life if you know what to do and what not to do and if you act quickly and calmly. If you are injured, do not lose your head and just call for help. Give the appropriate first aid and then seek medical assistance as soon as possible. KEEP CALM and BE GENTLE.

b. Your job is to fight! Fighting is your primary mission. Anything you can do to keep yourself and others in fighting condition is part of this mission. Luck is not the reason most casualties are able to return to their units to fight again; it is principally because they are given the appropriate first aid and excellent medical care. You can protect yourself and others by knowing first aid.

4. Vital Processes for Life

a. Blood Circulation. Blood circulation is a vital process for life. As the blood circulates through the body tissues, it provides them with the oxygen and food substances they must have to live and removes carbon dioxide and other waste products.. The blood is circulated through the body tissues by means of the heart and the blood vessels.

(1) *Heart.* The heart is essentially a hollow, muscular organ divided into a right and left side. It is located in the front part of the chest cage (*b*(3) below) between the lungs with about two-thirds of its mass to the left of the midline. The heart functions as a pump to circulate the blood through the blood vessels to various regions of the body. It contracts, thus forcing the blood from its chambers; then it relaxes, permitting its chambers to refill with blood. This cycle of contraction and relaxation, which is repeated continuously at a regular rhythmical rate, is called the heartbeat.

(2) *Blood vessels.* The blood vessels are the arteries, veins, and capillaries.

(*a*) *Arteries.* The arteries, which have thick, muscular walls, carry the richly oxygenated blood from the left side of the heart to all parts of the body. This blood is *bright* red because of its high oxygen content. It flows through the arteries in spurts which occur with each heartbeat. The arteries expand each time the heart forces blood into them and contract as the blood moves farther along the circulatory system. This cycle of expansion and contraction of the arteries is called the pulse. The normal average rate of the pulse is considered to be 60 to 80 beats per minute.

(*b*) *Veins.* The veins carry poorly oxygenated blood back to the heart from all parts of the body. This blood is *dark* red because of its low oxygen content. Its flow is not in spurts but continuous.

(*c*) *Capillaries.* The capillaries are the very small blood vessels interposed between the arteries and veins. Their walls are thin and very permeable, thus permitting the exchange of oxygen, food substances, carbon dioxide, et cetera, between the blood and the tissues. The capillary blood is *bright* or *dark* red. Its flow is very slow and sluggish.

b. Respiration (Inhalation and Exhalation). Respiration is a vital process for life. It is the means through which oxygen is taken into the body and carbon dioxide is expelled from the body. Oxygen is taken into the lungs as the air is inhaled; then it is picked up by blood vessels (*a*(2) above) and carried to all tissues throughout the body. Carbon dioxide is picked up by the blood vessels in the

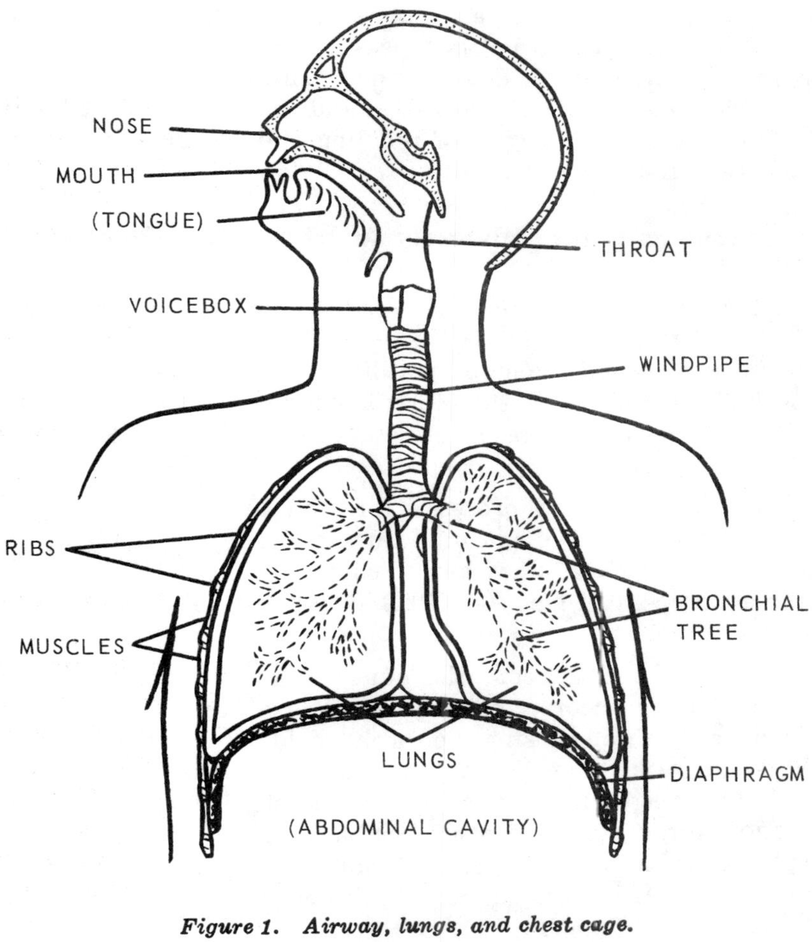

Figure 1. Airway, lungs, and chest cage.

tissues and carried to the lungs where it is deposited and expelled with exhalation. The process of respiration is accomplished by means of the airway, the lungs, and the chest cavity (fig 1).

(1) *Airway.* The airway is a canal through which air passes to and from the lungs. It consists of the nose, mouth, throat, voicebox, windpipe, and bronchial tree.

(2) *Lungs.* The lungs are two elastic organs made up of thousands of tiny air spaces and covered by an airtight membrane.

(3) *Chest cage.* The chest cage is formed by the muscle-connected ribs which join the spine in the back and the breastbone in the front. The top portion of the chest cage is closed by the structure of the neck, and the bottom portion is separated from the abdominal cavity by a large dome-shaped muscle called the diaphragm. The diaphragm and the rib muscles, which are under control of the respiratory center in the brain, automatically contract and relax, causing an increase and decrease in the size of the chest cage. When the chest cage increases and then decreases, the air pressure in the lungs is less and then more than the atmospheric pressure, thus causing air to rush in and out of the lungs to equalize the pressure. This cycle of inhaling and exhaling is repeated about 14 to 18 times per minute.

5. Conditions Which Adversely Affect the Vital Processes for Life

a. Lack of Oxygen. The vital processes for life (para 4) cannot continue without the intake of oxygen. The lack of oxygen not only will cause a casualty to stop breathing but also cause his heart to stop beating. You must, therefore, know how to clear a casualty's AIRWAY and restore respiration and heartbeat—LIFESAVING MEASURES A (chap 2).

b. Bleeding. The vital processes for life (para 4) cannot continue without an adequate volume of blood to carry oxygen to the tissues. You must, therefore, know how to control BLEEDING to prevent unnecessary loss of blood—LIFESAVING MEASURES B (chap 2).

c. Shock. Shock is a condition of acute circulatory failure. Shock which remains uncorrected may result in death even though the injury or condition causing the shock would not be otherwise fatal. Shock can result from many causes such as loss of blood, loss of fluid from deep burns, expansion of the blood vessels, pain, and reaction to the sight of a wound or blood. You must know how to apply shock CONTROLS, as a casualty's chances of survival are much greater if he does not develop this condition—LIFESAVING MEASURES C (chap 2).

d. Infection. Recovery from a severe injury or healing of a wound is greatly dependent upon how well the wound was protected from contamination initially. Infection results from the multiplication and growth of germs which invade a wound or a break in the skin by contamination. Since germs are in the air and on the skin and clothing, some of them will get into every wound immediately. The objective is to keep additional germs out of the wound. You must, therefore, know how to apply DRESSINGS and bandages to protect the wound from contamination—LIFESAVING MEASURES D (chap 2).

6. First Aid Supplies

The supplies which will be available for your use in giving first aid will depend upon where you are at the time.

a. Personal First Aid Items. You are issued a first aid case containing two packets for your personal use (fig 2). One packet contains a sterile dressing with attached bandages for use on a wound, and the other packet contains two envelopes of sodium chloride-sodium bicarbonate mixture for consumption if you are burned. You must have this case of items with you at all times. As a good soldier, you check your individual weapon each day; you should be just as careful about checking your first aid case to insure that the proper first aid items are in it. When applying first aid to a casualty, remember to use *his* first aid items first; you may need *yours* later on!

b. General Purpose First Aid Kit. This first aid kit is carried in all vehicles. For a list of items which it contains, see appendix B.

c. Airplane First Aid Kit. This first aid kit is carried in aircraft. For a list of items which it contains, see appendix B.

d. Emergency Medical Treatment Unit—Phase I. In the event of a nuclear attack while in garrison, the number of casualties that may result could overload existing medical facilities during the first few hours following the attack. Medical personnel will treat casualties according to established priorities dictated by the type of injury of each casualty. Under these conditions, you may have to take care of yourself or others around you until trained medical personnel can get to you. The medical supplies which you will need have been packaged and placed in buildings where you work or live so that they will be readily available. These boxes are clearly labeled *Emergency Medical Treatment Unit—Phase I* (fig 3). This Phase I Unit contains seven component packs: four wound packs, two burn packs, and one fracture pack. For a list of items in each type of pack, see appendix B. Familiarize yourself with the loca-

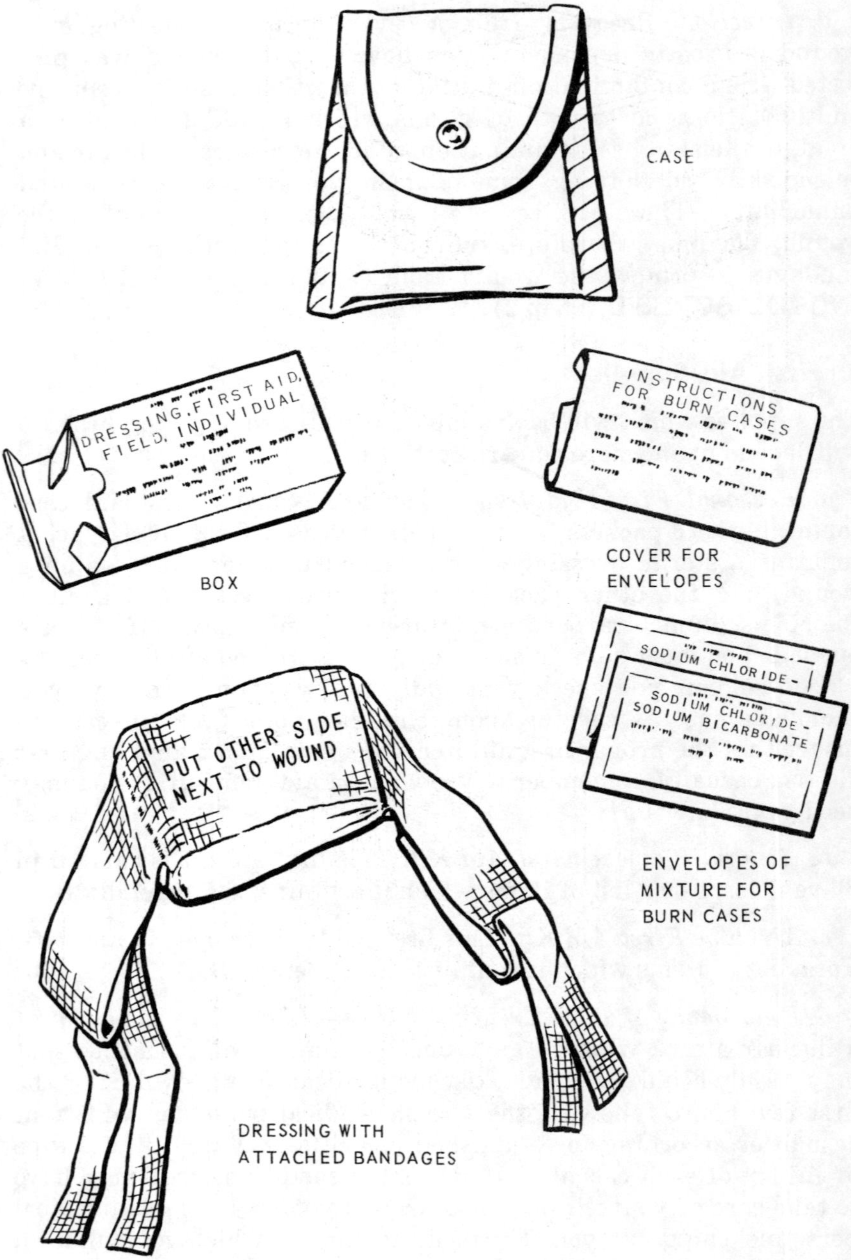

Figure 2. First aid case and contents.

tion of the Phase I Units in your area, the contents of each pack contained in the unit, and how to use this material to save your life or the lives of other persons who may not be able to help them-

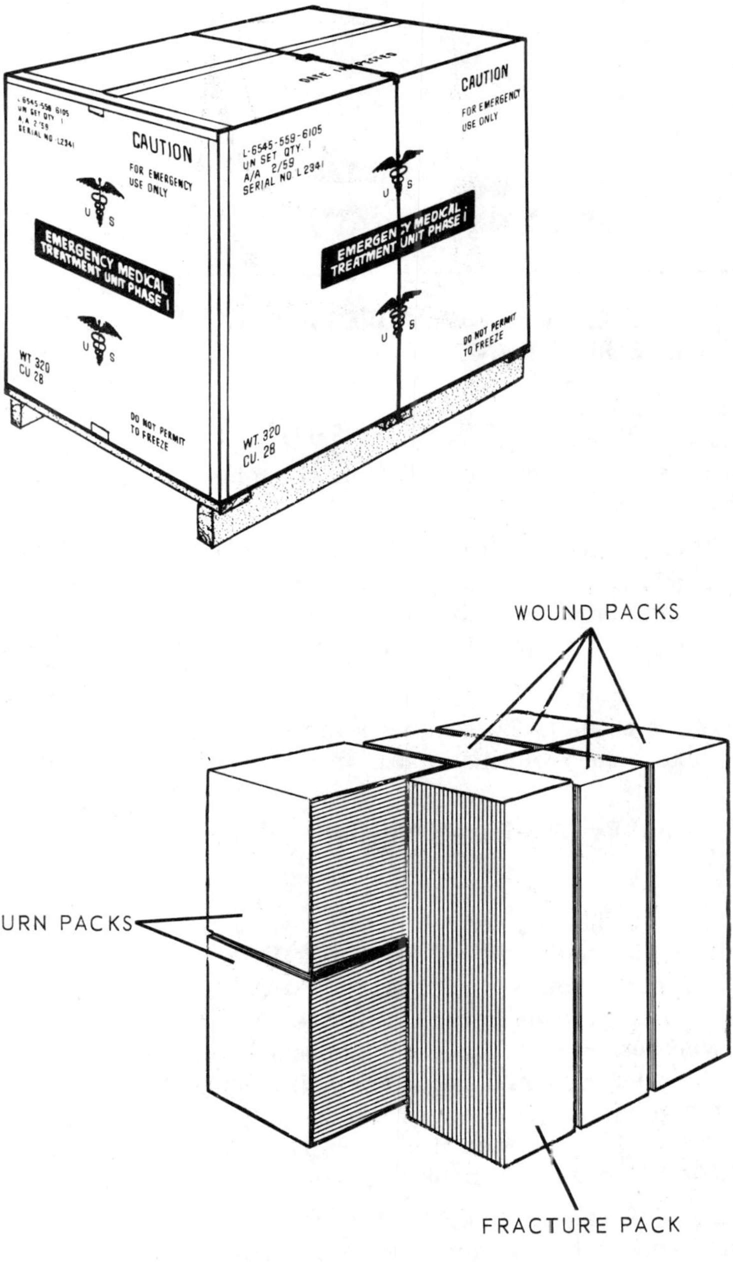

Figure 3. Emergency Medical Treatment Unit—Phase I.

selves. Succeeding chapters in this manual will tell you how to use most of the items contained in the Phase I Unit. Items not discussed in this manual should be used only by persons who have received special instructions in how to use them.

CHAPTER 2

LIFESAVING MEASURES A B C D

Section I. LIFESAVING MEASURES A: CLEAR THE AIRWAY AND RESTORE BREATHING AND HEARTBEAT AS NECESSARY

7. Upper Airway—Clear Immediately!

In order for air to flow to and from the lungs, the airway must be unobstructured.

a. To clear the casualty's upper airway, turn his head to one side and quickly remove from his mouth any vomitus, mucus, or debris by running your fingers behind his lower teeth and over the back of his tongue. This process should not take more than a second or two.

b. If the casualty is wearing removable dentures (full or partial), take them from his mouth and put them in his pocket.

8. Artificial Respiration—If Needed, Administer Immediately!

a. General.

(1) If a casualty stops breathing, you must give him artificial respiration immediately. SECONDS COUNT! Be calm! Think and act! The sooner you begin the artificial respiration, the more likely you are to succeed in restoring his breathing. If you are in doubt as to whether or not the casualty is breathing, do not waste valuable seconds but give him artificial respiration, as it can do no harm to a person who is breathing. If the casualty is breathing, you can ordinarily feel and see his chest moving or feel and hear air being expelled by putting your hand or ear close to his mouth and nose.

(2) If a casualty has no heartbeat, he must also be given closed-chest heart massage immediately as described in paragraph 9. If two persons are available, one can give artificial respiration while the other one gives closed-chest heart massage. If you are the only person available, you must perform both measures, alternating them as prescribed in paragraph 9*c*(3) (*c*).

(3) There are two primary methods for administering artifi-

cial respiration: the mouth-to-mouth method and the chest-pressure arm-lift method. The mouth-to-mouth method is the preferred one; however it cannot be used if the casualty has a crushed face or is in a toxic environment. In the case of crushed face or the absence of a mask equipped with a resuscitation device, the chest-pressure arm-lift method must be used. The mouth-to-mouth method may be modified somewhat and referred to as the mouth-to-nose method and as the mask-to-mouth method used in a toxic environment (para 52*d*).

b. Mouth-to-Mouth (Nose) Method. In this method of artificial respiration, you inflate the casualty's lungs with air from your lungs. This can be accomplished by blowing air into either his mouth or his nose. The mouth is the preferred airway opening except for a casualty who has a severe jaw fracture or mouth wound or whose jaws are tightly closed by spasms. For this casualty the nose must be used. The mouth-to-mouth (nose) method is performed as follows:

(1) Clear the casualty's upper airway (para 7).

(2) Position the casualty on his back.

(3) Position the casualty's head with his face up and place a rolled blanket or some other similar object under his *shoulders* so that his head will drop back (fig 4). If such an object is not immediately available, tilt his head back so that the neck is extended and the head is in a chin-up position. This position helps to enlarge the airway passage.

(4) Adjust the casualty's lower jaw to a jutting-out position (fig 5). This positioning moves the base of the tongue farther away from the back of the throat, thus enlarging the airway passage to the lungs. It may be accomplished by either the thumb jaw-lift or the two-hand jaw-lift.

(*a*) *Thumb jaw-lift.* This is ordinarily the choice method for adjusting the jaw unless the nature of the injury prevents its use. Place the thumb in the casualty's mouth, grasp the lower jaw firmly, and lift it forward (a, fig 5). Do not attempt to hold or depress the tongue.

(*b*) *Two-hand jaw-lift.* In case the casualty's jaws are so tightly closed that the thumb cannot be inserted into the mouth, the two-hand jaw-lift is used. Grasping the angles of the lower jaw with both hands just below the ear lobes, lift the jaw forcibly forward; then open the lips by pushing the lower lip toward the chin with the thumbs (b, fig 5).

(5) Continuing to hold the casualty's jaw forward, seal the airway opening (nose or mouth) which is not to be used when

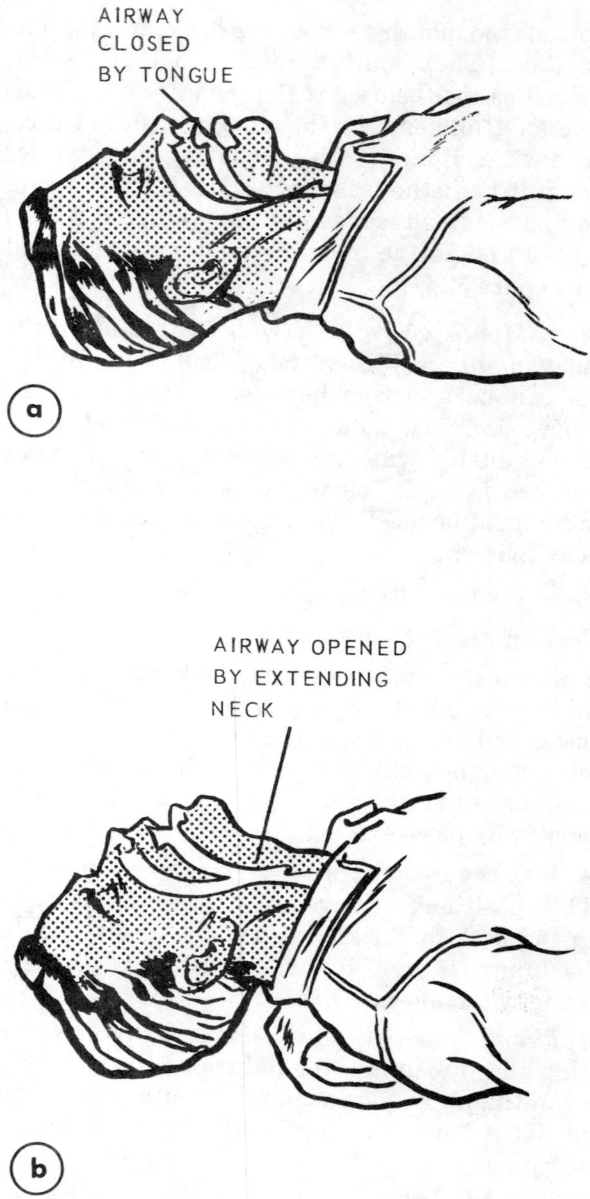

Figure 4. Shoulder raised and head tilted back in chin-up position.

inflating his lungs. The seal must be secure to prevent leakage of air. If the nose is to be sealed, pinch it shut with your free hand (a, fig 6) or press your cheek firmly against it (b fig 6). If the mouth is to be sealed, firmly close the lips with two fingers placed lengthwise. (If the casualty is an infant or small child, both the mouth and nose are left open ((6) (*a*) below).)

(a)

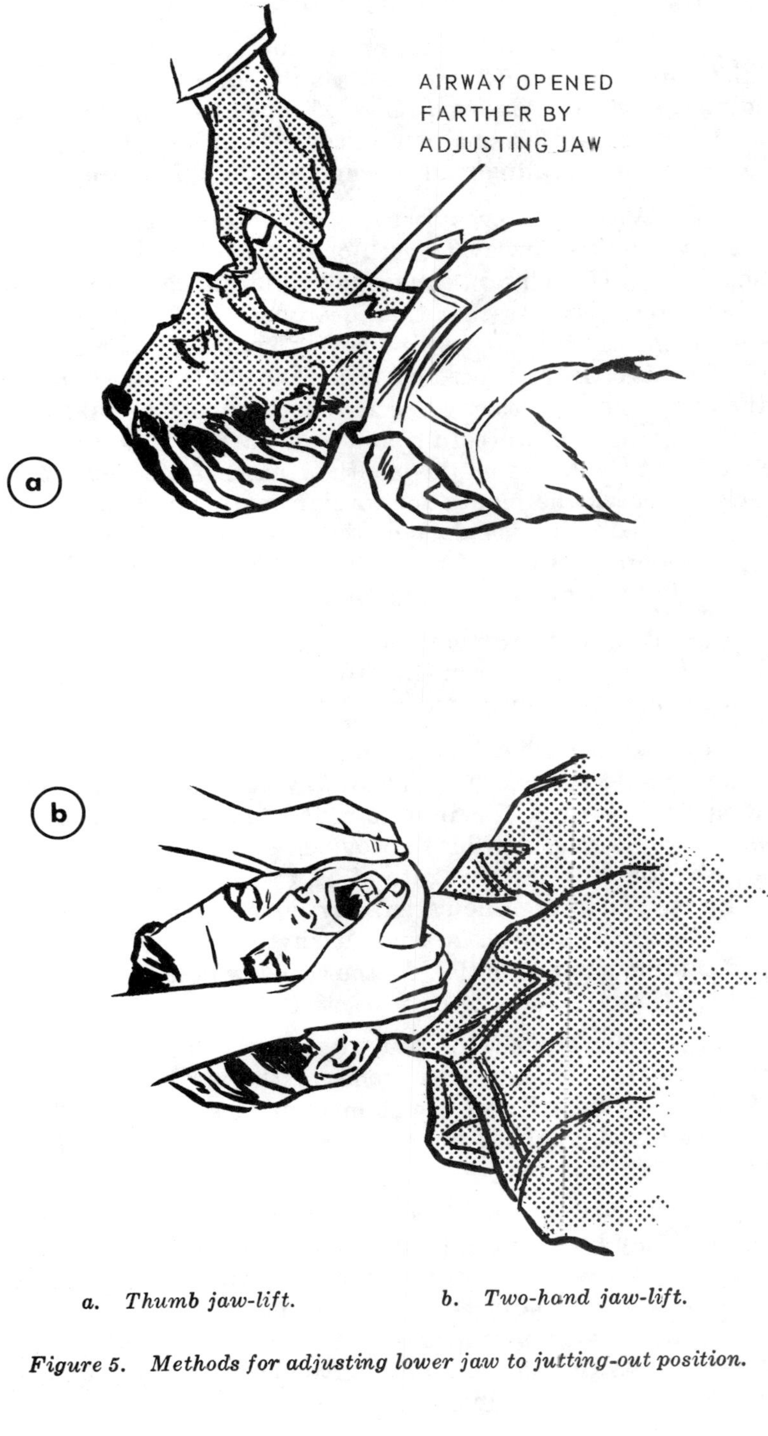

(b)

a. Thumb jaw-lift. *b. Two-hand jaw-lift.*

Figure 5. Methods for adjusting lower jaw to jutting-out position.

(6) Administer artificial respiration as follows:

(*a*) Take a deep breath, open your mouth wide, and make an airtight seal around the casualty's mouth (fig 6) or nose, depending upon which one you have left open ((5) above). (If the patient is an infant or small child, cover both his nose and mouth with your mouth, sealing your lips against the skin of his face.)

(*b*) With your eyes focused on the casualty's chest, blow forcefully into his airway (mouth or nose) unless he is an infant or small child. (Into infants and small children, blow small puffs of air from your cheeks rather than deep breaths from your lungs.) Rising of the casualty's chest indicates that the air is reaching his lungs. In this case the procedure is continued ((*c*) and (*d*) below). If the chest does not rise, corrective action must be taken. First, hold the jaw up more forcefully and blow harder, making sure that the air is not leaking from the mouth or nose. If the chest still does not rise, recheck the mouth for foreign matter and, if necessary, turn the casualty on his side and strike him between the shoulders with considerable force, repeatedly if necessary, to dislodge obstruction in the airway; then inflate his lungs.

(*c*) Remove your mouth from the casualty's airway opening and listen for the return of air from his lungs. If the casualty's exhalation is noisy, elevate his jaw more.

(*d*) After each exhalation of air from the casualty's lungs, blow another deep breath into his airway. Make the first five to ten breaths deep (except for infants and small children) and give them at a rapid rate in order to provide fast reoxygenation. Thereafter, give the breaths at a rate of 12 to 20 per minute until the casualty is able to breathe satisfactorily for himself or until you are positive life is gone. A smooth rhythm is desired but split second timing is not essential. As the casualty attempts to breathe, adjust the timing of your efforts to assist him.

1. After a period of resuscitation the casualty's abdomen may bulge. This indicates that some of the air is going into his stomach. Since inflation of the stomach makes it more difficult to inflate the lungs, apply gentle pressure to the abdomen with your hand between inflations.

2. If your breathing at the start has been very deep and rapid, you may become faint, tingle, or even lose consciousness if you persist. After administering the first five to ten deep, rapid breaths, you should adjust your breathing to a rate of 12 to 20 times a minute with only moderate increase in normal volume so that you will be able to continue to give artificial respiration for a long period without temporary ill effects. (If you becomes dis-

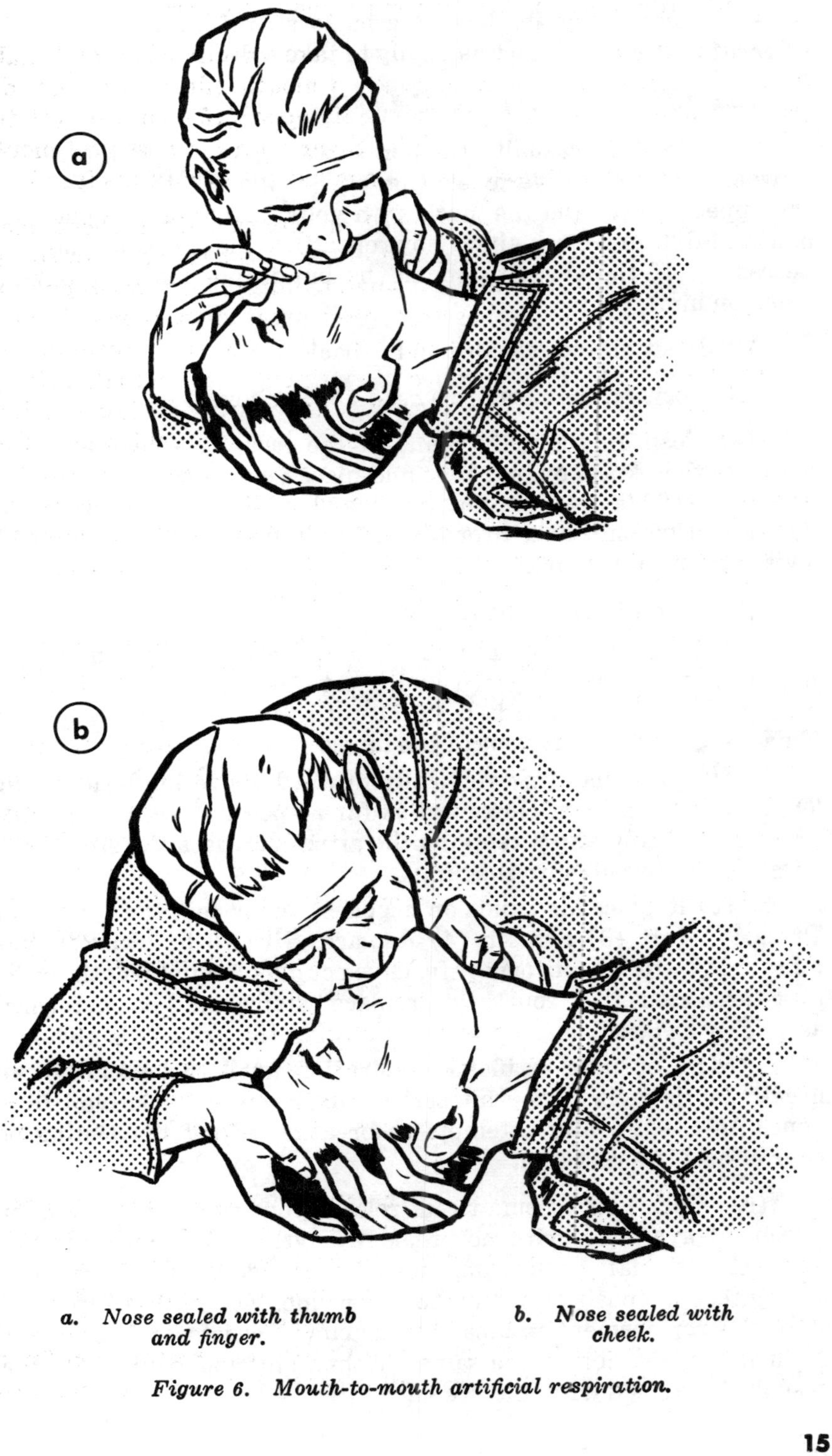

a. Nose sealed with thumb and finger.

b. Nose sealed with cheek.

Figure 6. Mouth-to-mouth artificial respiration.

tressed from giving shallow breaths to an infant or small child, interrupt your rhythm occasionally to take a deep breath.)

c. Chest-Pressure Arm-Lift Method.

(1) Clear the casualty's upper airway (para 7). If the patient is wearing a protective mask (fig 7), quickly lift the mask, clear the upper airway and the mask with your fingers, and replace the mask. Maintain a clear airway by repeating this procedure later, if necessary. If the casualty should be but is not masked, put his mask on him.

(2) Position the casualty on his back.

(3) Position the casualty's head (*b*(3) above).

(4) Position yourself: Stand at the casualty's head and face his feet; then kneel on one knee and place your opposite foot to the other side of his head and against his shoulder to steady it (a, fig 7). If you become uncomfortable after a period of time, quickly switch to the other knee.

(5) Administer artificial respiration:

(*a*) Grasping the casualty's hands and holding them over his lower ribs, rock forward and exert steady, uniform pressure almost directly downward (b, fig 7) until you meet firm resistance. This pressure forces air out of the lungs.

(*b*) Lift his arms vertically upward above his head (c, fig 7); then stretch them backward as far as possible (d, fig 7). This process of lifting and stretching the arms increases the size of the chest and draws air into the lungs.

(*c*) Replace his hands on his chest and repeat the cycle: (1) Press (2) Lift (3) Stretch (4) Replace. Give 10 to 12 cycles per minute at a steady uniform rate. Give counts of equal length to the first three steps. The fourth or "replace" step should be performed as quickly as possible.

(*d*) Continue artificial respiration until the casualty can breathe satisfactorily for himself or until you are positive life is gone. As the casualty attempts to breathe, adjust the timing of your efforts to assist him.

(6) When you become tired, release your position to another person, if available, with no break in rhythm. Continuing to administer artificial respiration, move to one side while the replacement takes his position from the other side. During the "stretch" step, the replacement grasps the casualty's wrists and continues artificial respiration in the same rhythm, shifting his grip to the casualty's hands during the "replace" step.

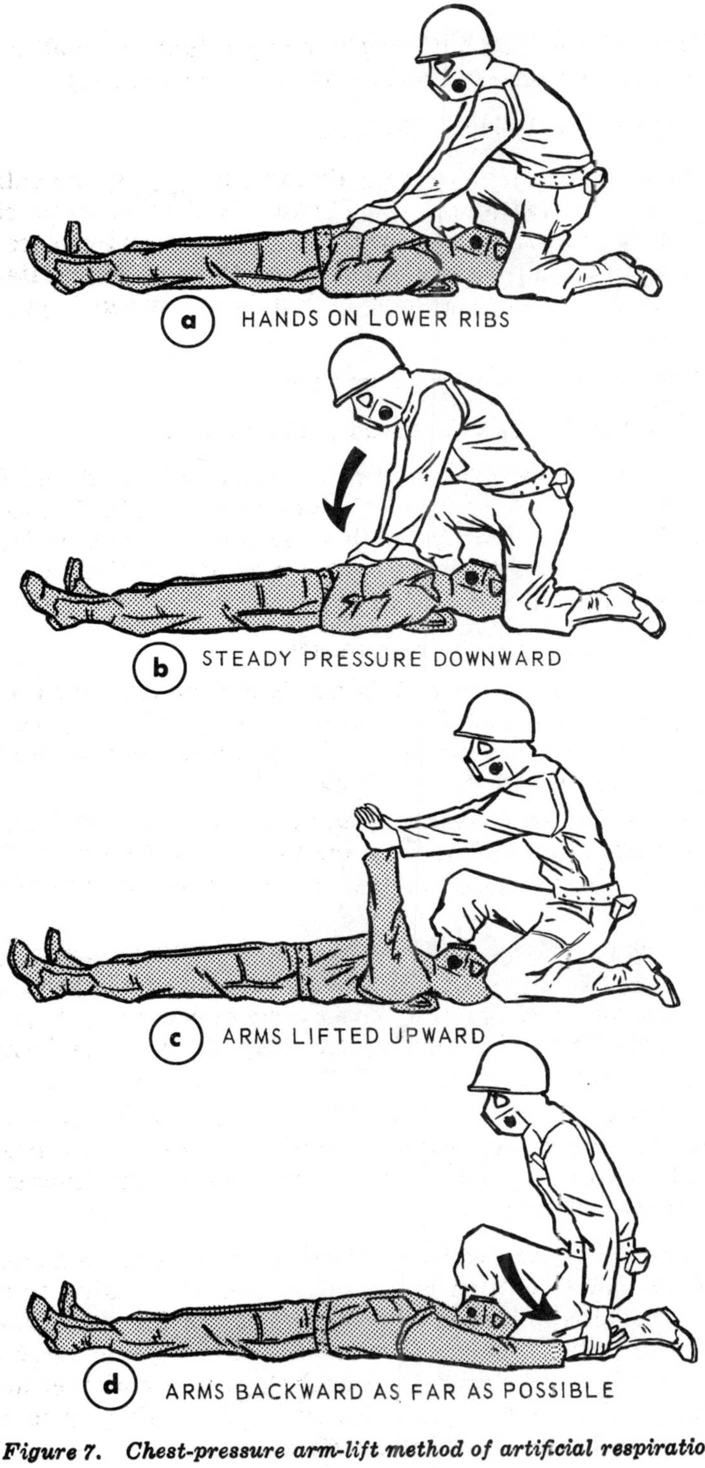

Figure 7. Chest-pressure arm-lift method of artificial respiration.

9. Closed-Chest Heart Massage—If Needed, Administer Immediately!

a. General. If a casualty's heart stops beating, you must give him closed-chest heart massage as well as artificial respiration immediately. SECONDS COUNT! Stoppage of the heart is soon followed by cessation of respiration unless this occurred first. Be calm! Think and act! When a casualty's heart has stopped, he has no pulse at all (para 4*a*(2) (*a*)) ; he is unconscious and limp, and the pupils of his eyes are open wide. To determine the presence or absence of the casualty's pulse, place the tips of your fingers on his neck to the side of his windpipe as illustrated in figure 8. If you do not detect a pulse immediately, do not waste time checking further; start heart massage at once. Furthermore, if you find the casualty's pulse to be very weak and irregular, you must give him closed-chest heart massage and artificial respiration, as these signs indicate ineffective beats of the heart and precede heart stoppage.

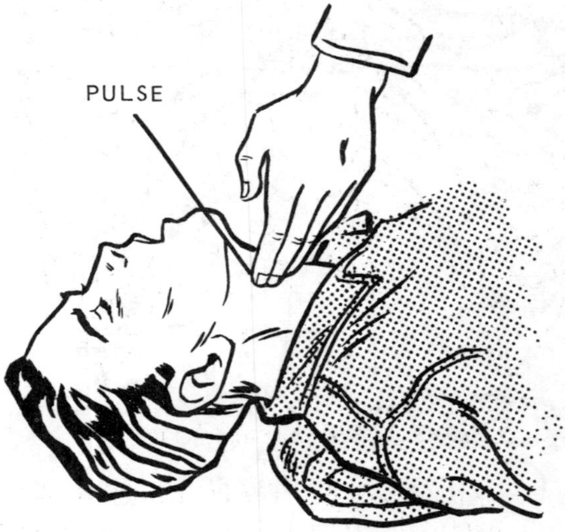

Figure 8. Placement of fingers to detect pulse.

b. General Principles of Closed-Chest Heart Massage.

(1) Closed-chest heart massage is the rhythmical compression of the heart without surgically opening the chest. It is designed to provide artificial circulation in order to keep blood flowing to the brain and other organs until the heart begins to beat normally again. This is not the same as open-chest heart massage, in which the chest wall is cut open and the heart itself is compressed directly by hand.

(2) The heart is located between the breastbone and the spine (fig 9). Pressure on the breastbone pushes the heart against the spine, thus forcing blood out of the heart into the arteries. Release of pressure allows the heart to refill with blood.

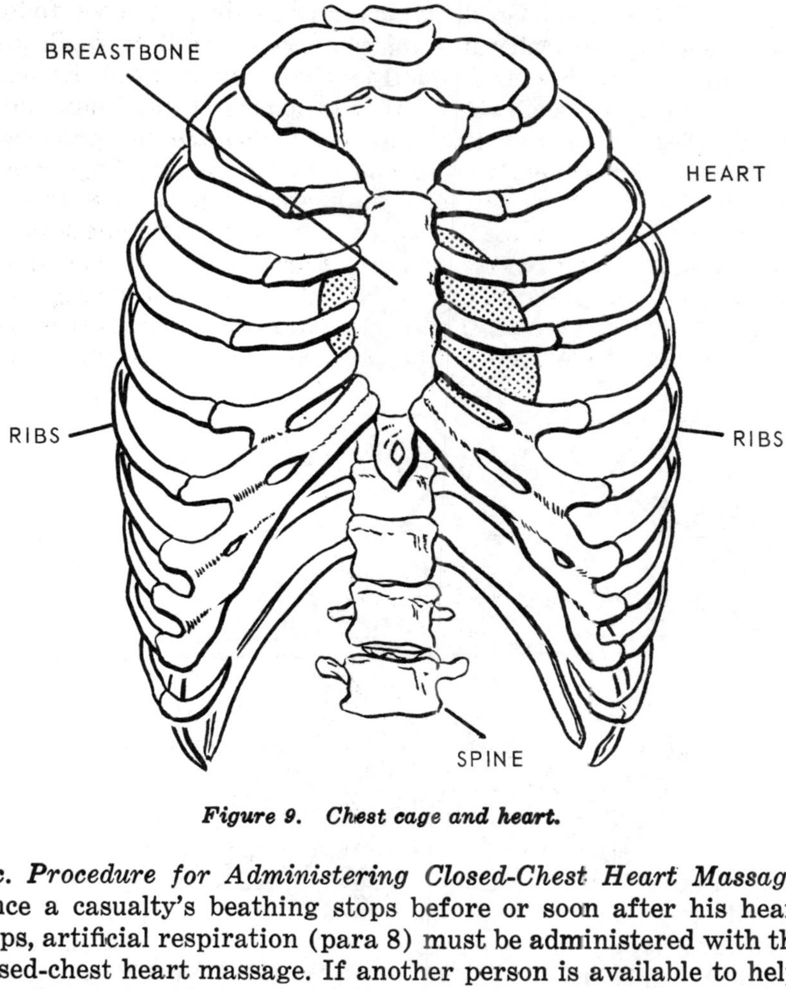

Figure 9. Chest cage and heart.

c. Procedure for Administering Closed-Chest Heart Massage. Since a casualty's beathing stops before or soon after his heart stops, artificial respiration (para 8) must be administered with the closed-chest heart massage. If another person is available to help, one of you should give heart massage while the outer one gives artificial respiration (fig 10). The two of you should coordinate your efforts so that one is not blowing into casualty's airway at the same time that the other one is pressing on his breastbone. If you must administer first aid alone, alternate these measures as described in (3) (*c*) below.

(1) Prepare the casualty for the mouth-to-mouth (nose) method of artificial respiration (para 8*b*). The surface on which the casualty is placed MUST BE SOLID. A litter, the floor, or the

ground is adequate. A bed or couch is too flexible.

(2) Position yourself:

(*a*) Kneel at a right angle to the casualty's chest so that you can use your weight to apply pressure on his breastbone (fig 10).

(*b*) Place the heel of one hand on the LOWER half of the breastbone. Spread and raise your fingers so you can apply pressure without pressing the ribs. Place your other hand on top of the first. (If the casualty is a child, omit placing the second hand over the first. If the patient is an infant, place only the fingertips of one hand on the breastbone.)

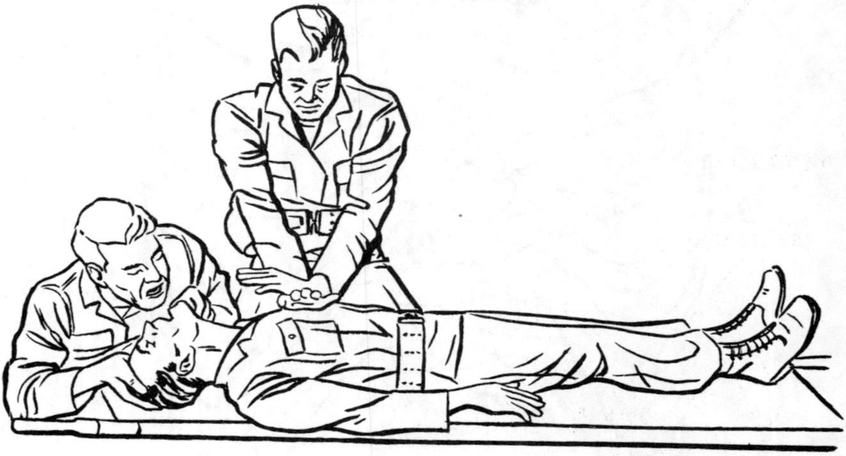

Figure 10. Closed-chest heart massage and mouth-to-mouth artificial respiration when two persons are available.

(3) Administer closed-heart massage:

(*a*) With your hands in the correct position ((2) (*b*) above) and your arms straight, lean forward to bring your shoulders directly above the casualty's breastbone; then press straight downward. Apply enough pressure to push the breastbone down 1½ to 2 inches (fig 11). Too much pressure may fracture the casualty's ribs; therefore do NOT push the breastbone down more than 2 inches. (If the casualty is a child, press his breastbone lightly with only one hand. If the casualty is an infant, press the breastbone lightly with your fingers.)

(*b*) Release the pressure immediately, lifting the hands slightly (fig 12).

(*c*) Repeat the press-release cycle 60 to 80 times per minute. After a few minutes, check for a pulse by placing your fingers on the casualty's neck as illustrated in figure 8 or by looking for

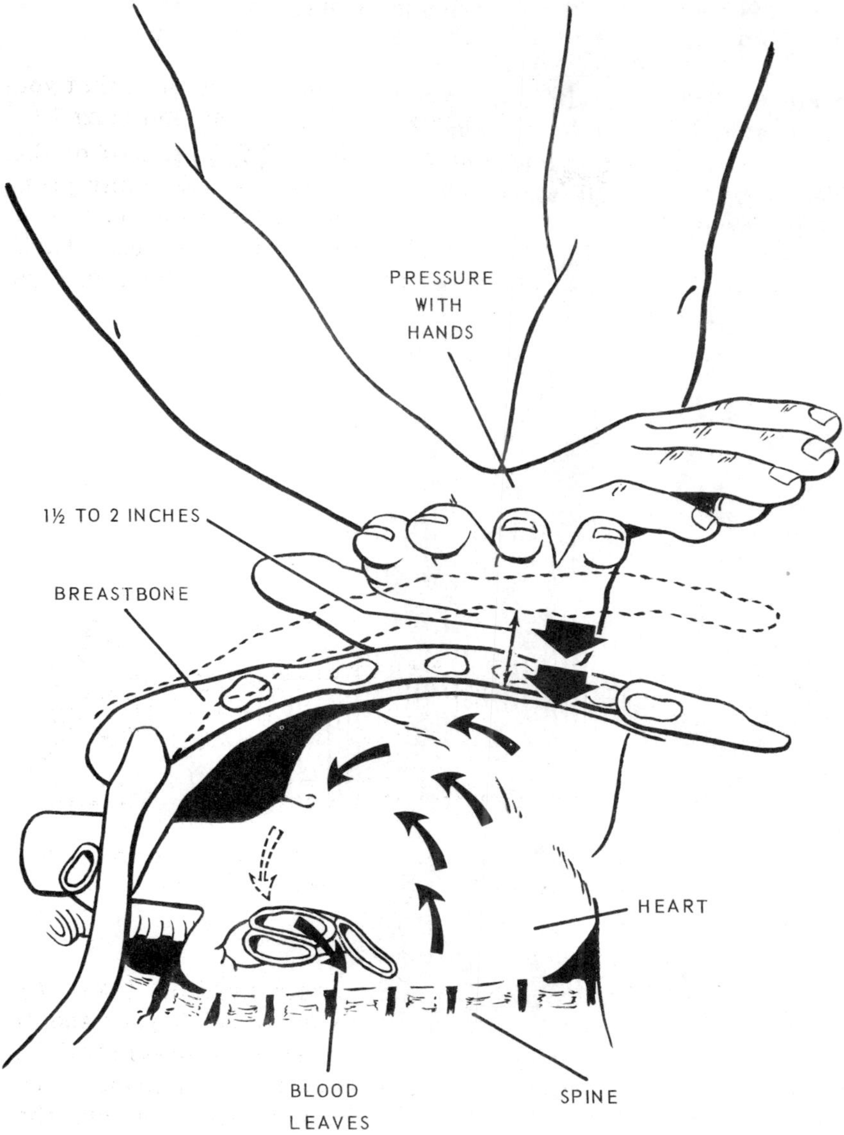

Figure 11. Blood forced out of the heart into the arteries by application of pressure on the breastbone.

movement at this spot on his neck. If only a feeble, irregular pulse or no pulse can be detected, elevate the casualty's legs about 6 inches above the level of his head to help the return of blood to his heart. Continue the heart massage and the mouth-to-mouth resuscitation until the casualty is able to function without assistance, until you are relieved, or until you are positive life is gone. If performing alone, give four or five cycles of heart massage then one cycle of artificial respiration. It may be necessary for you to perform these resuscitative measures a long time after you feel the heavy effects of bodily discomfort and fatigue. Cessation of resuscitative measures must rest on the judgment of the most qualified person available and not on the state of discomfort of the resuscitator.

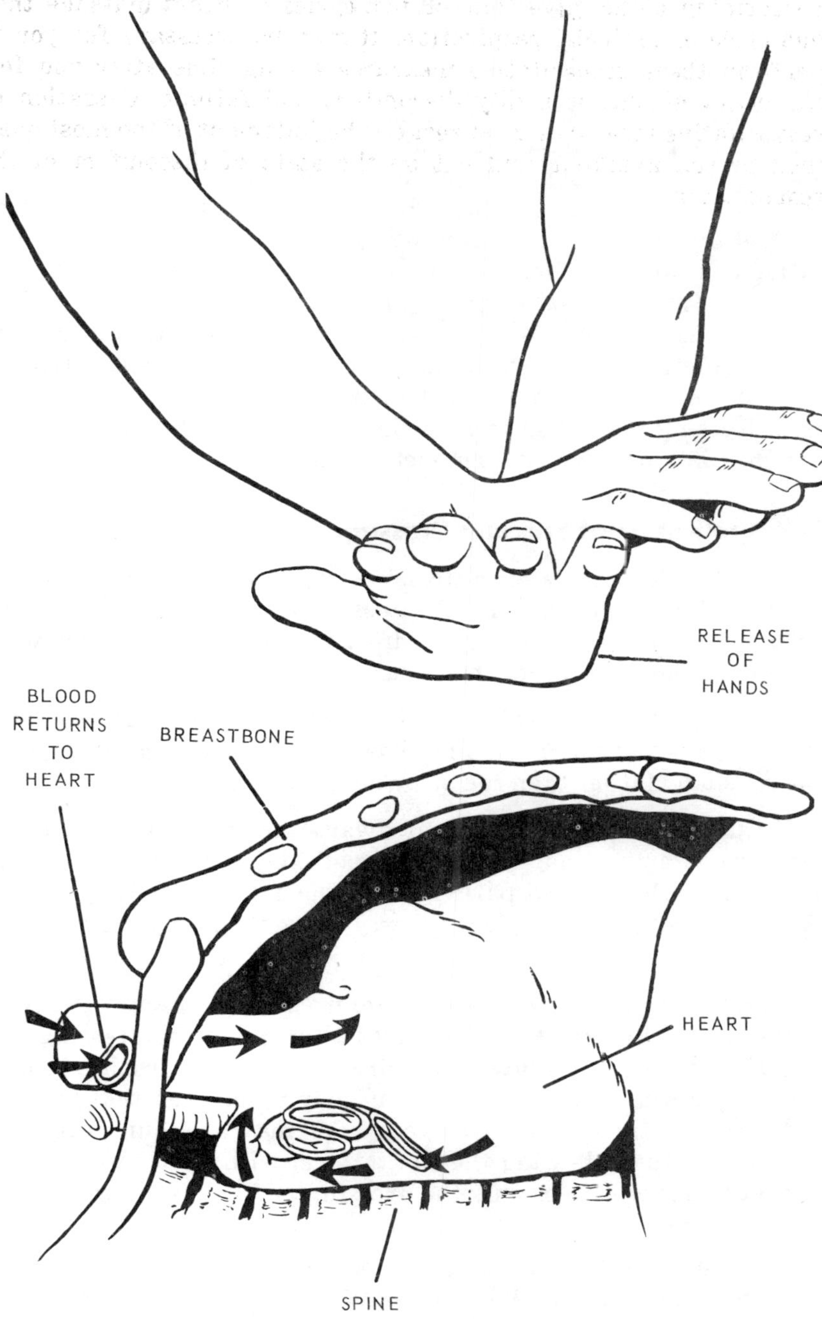

Figure 12 *Release of pressure to allow the heart to refill with blood.*

Section II. LIFESAVING MEASURES B: STOP THE BLEEDING

10. General

Wounds are the most common conditions needing first aid. Uncontrolled bleeding from wounds causes shock and finally death. You must, therefore, apply appropriate first aid measures to stop bleeding. The use of the pressure dressing (para 11) is the choice method for the control of bleeding in an emergency situation. Elevation of a wounded limb (para 11*c*(1)) and application of digital pressure (para 11*c*(2)) should also be used, as appropriate, in conjunction with the pressure dressing. The application of a tourniquet (para 12) is another method to control bleeding from a limb. A tourniquet should not be used, however, unless the pressure dressing has failed to stop the bleeding, as the casualty may lose the limb to which a tourniquet has been applied.

11. Application of Pressure Dressing

The application of a sterile dressing with pressure to a bleeding wound helps clot formation, compresses the open blood vessels, and protects the wound from further invasion of germs. The following procedure should be used when a person is wounded.

a. Look for more than one wound. For example, a missile may have come out at another point. The wound where a missile comes out is usually larger than the one where it enters.

b. Cut the clothing and lift it away from the wound to avoid further contamination. Tearing the clothing might result in rough handling of the injured part. Do not touch the wound; keep it as clean as possible. If it is already dirty, leave it that way. Do not try to clean it in any way.

c. Cover the wound with a first aid dressing and apply pressure to the wound by use of the bandages attached to the dressing (fig 13). If additional pressure is required to stop the bleeding, apply another pressure dressing or place your hand over the dressing and press hard. Pressure from your hand may be required for 5 to 10 minutes, thus allowing the clot to form with sufficient strength to hold with the help of only the dressing and bandages when your hand is removed.

(1) Frequently, bleeding can be lessened by raising the injured part above the level of the heart (c, fig. 13). Elevation is not used if there is a broken bone in the injured part. Moving an unsplinted fracture causes pain, can increase shock, and may further damage nerves, muscles, and blood vessels.

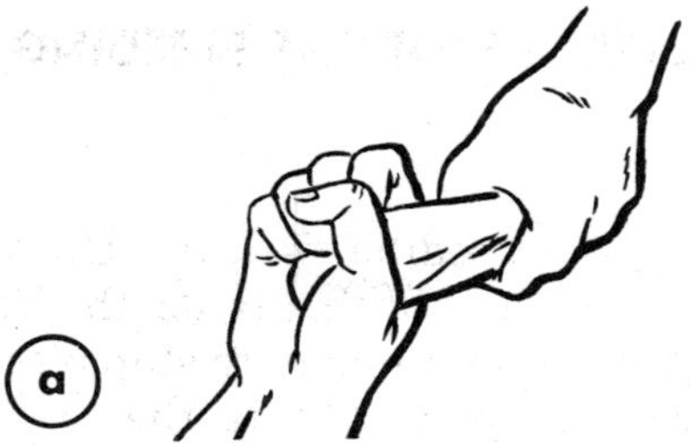

(a) REMOVE WRAPPED DRESSING WITH ATTACHED BANDAGES FROM BOX AND PLASTIC BAG; THEN TWIST TO BREAK PAPER WRAPPER.

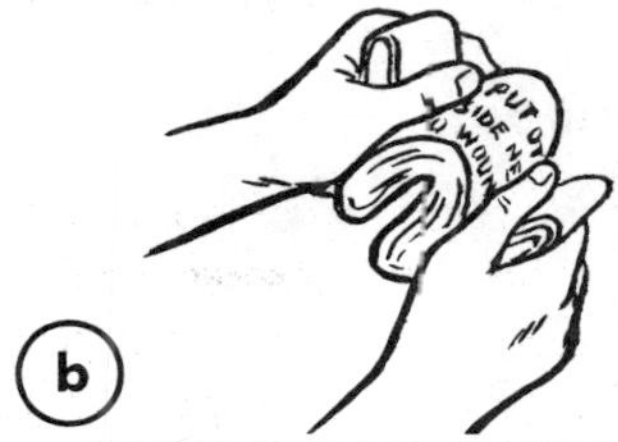

(b) GRASP FOLDED BANDAGES WITH HANDS, BEING CAREFUL NOT TO TOUCH SIDE OF DRESSING WHICH GOES NEXT TO WOUND.

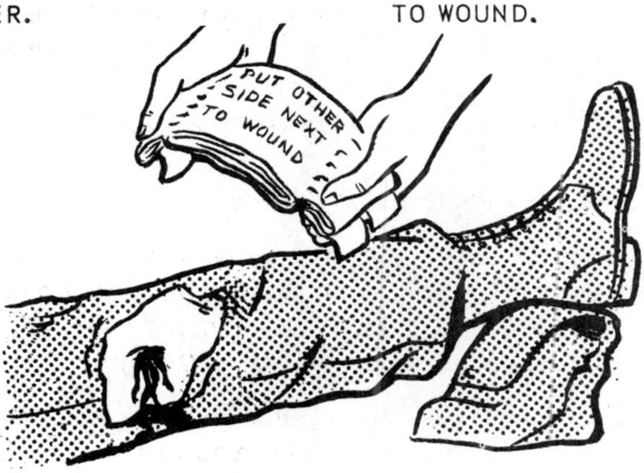

(c) CONTINUING TO HOLD FOLDED BANDAGES, PULL DRESSING OPEN.

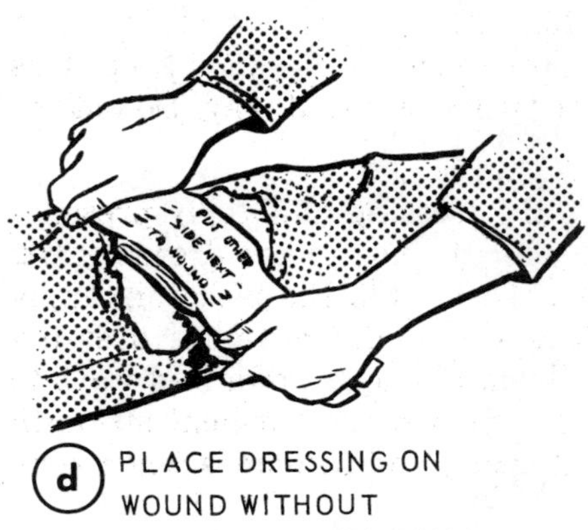

(d) PLACE DRESSING ON WOUND WITHOUT ALLOWING IT TO TOUCH ANYTHING ELSE.

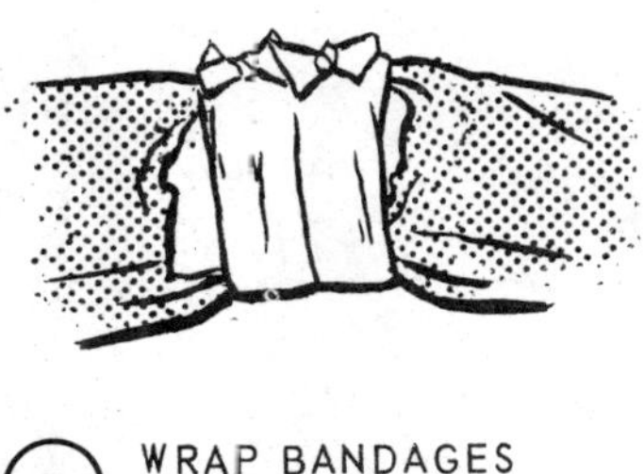

(e) WRAP BANDAGES AROUND THE PART AND TIE THE ENDS SECURELY.

Figure 13. Application of pressure dressing.

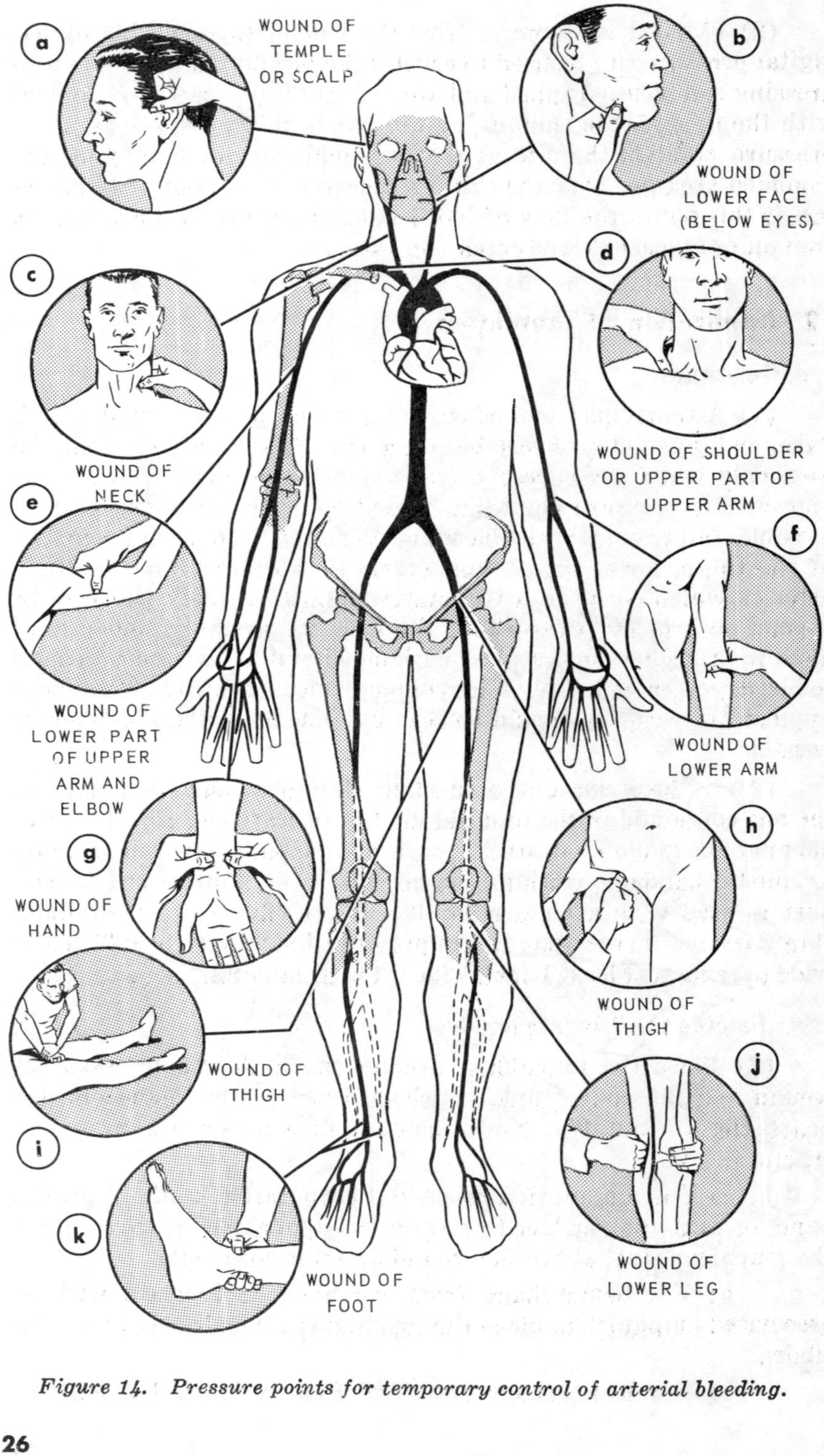

Figure 14. Pressure points for temporary control of arterial bleeding.

(2) If blood is spurting from the wound (arterial bleeding), digital pressure can be used to control the bleeding until a pressure dressing can be unwrapped and applied. Digital pressure is applied with the fingers, the thumbs, or the hands to a pressure point. A pressure point is the site at which a main artery supplying the wounded area lies near the skin surface and over a bone. By pressing at this point, the flow of blood from the heart to the wound is shut off or at least slowed down (fig 14).

12. Application of Tourniquet

a. General.

(1) A tourniquet is a constricting band placed around a limb (arm or leg) to stop severe bleeding (fig 15 and 16). It should be used only when pressure over the wound area, pressure over the appropriate pressure point, and elevation of the wounded part, if possible, fail to control the bleeding. Bleeding from a major artery of the thigh, lower leg or upper arm or bleeding from multiple arteries which occur in a traumatic amputation may prove to be beyond control by pressure. If the first aid dressing under hard hand pressure becomes soaked with blood and the wound continues to bleed, you should apply a tourniquet. Once a tourniquet has been applied, the casualty should be seen by a medical officer as soon as possible.

(2) In the absence of a specially designed tourniquet such as the one contained in the first aid kit for aircraft (fig 15), a tourniquet may be made from strong, soft, pliable material such as gauze or muslin bandage, clothing, or kerchiefs. An improvised tourniquet is used with a rigid stick-like object (fig 16). To minimize skin damage, insure that the improvised tourniquet is sufficiently wide to remain at least 1-inch wide after tightening.

b. Placing the Tourniquet.

(1) Place the tourniquet around the limb and between the wound and the body trunk, which is between the wound and the heart (fig 15 and 16). Never place it directly over a wound or fracture.

(*a*) For amputation or partial amputation of the foot, leg, hand, or arm and for bleeding from the upper arm or thigh, place the tourniquet just above the wound or amputation site.

(*b*) For hemorrhage from the hand or forearm with no associated amputation, place the tourniquet immediately above the elbow.

(*c*) For hemorrhage from the foot or lower leg with no

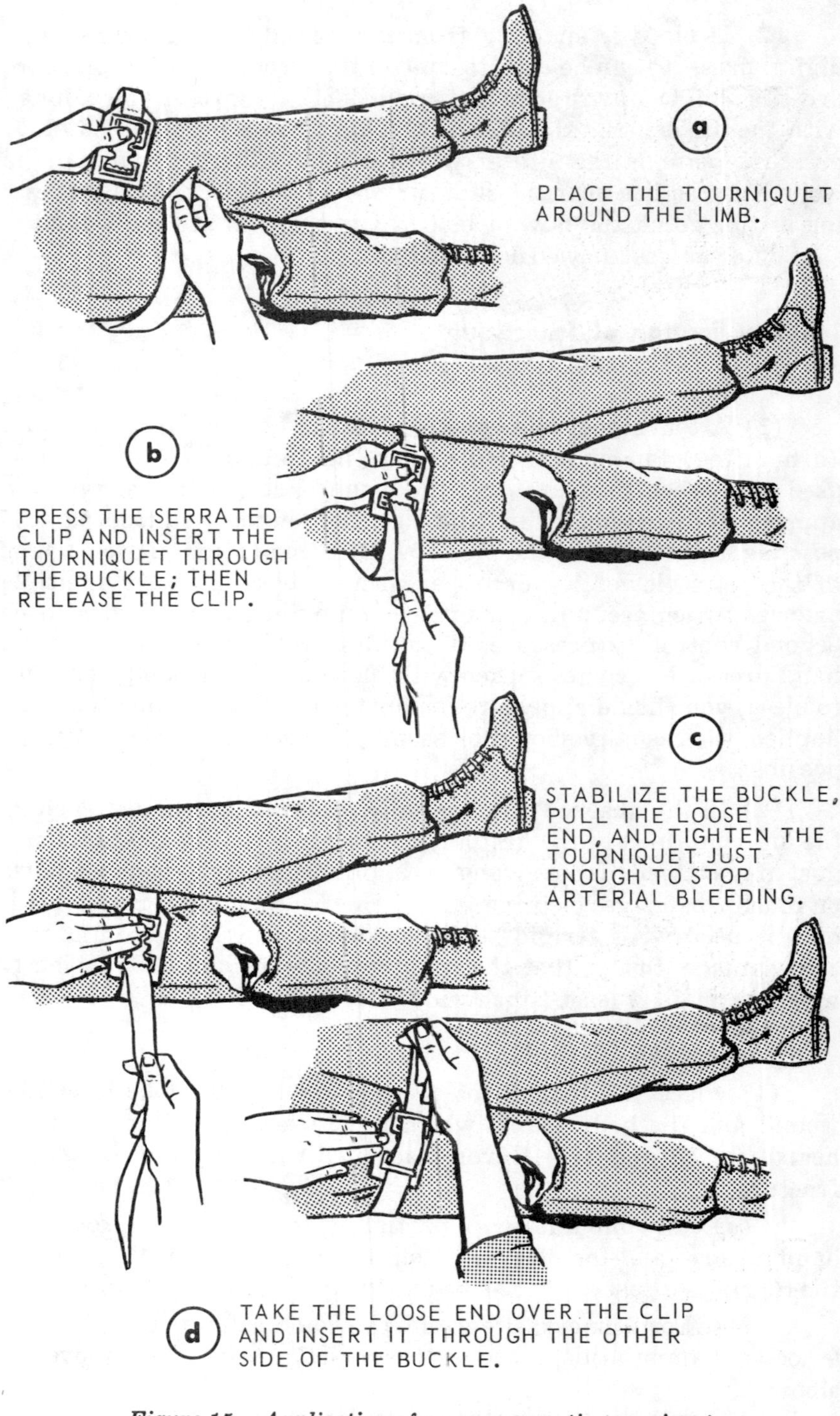

Figure 15. Application of a nonpneumatic tourniquet.

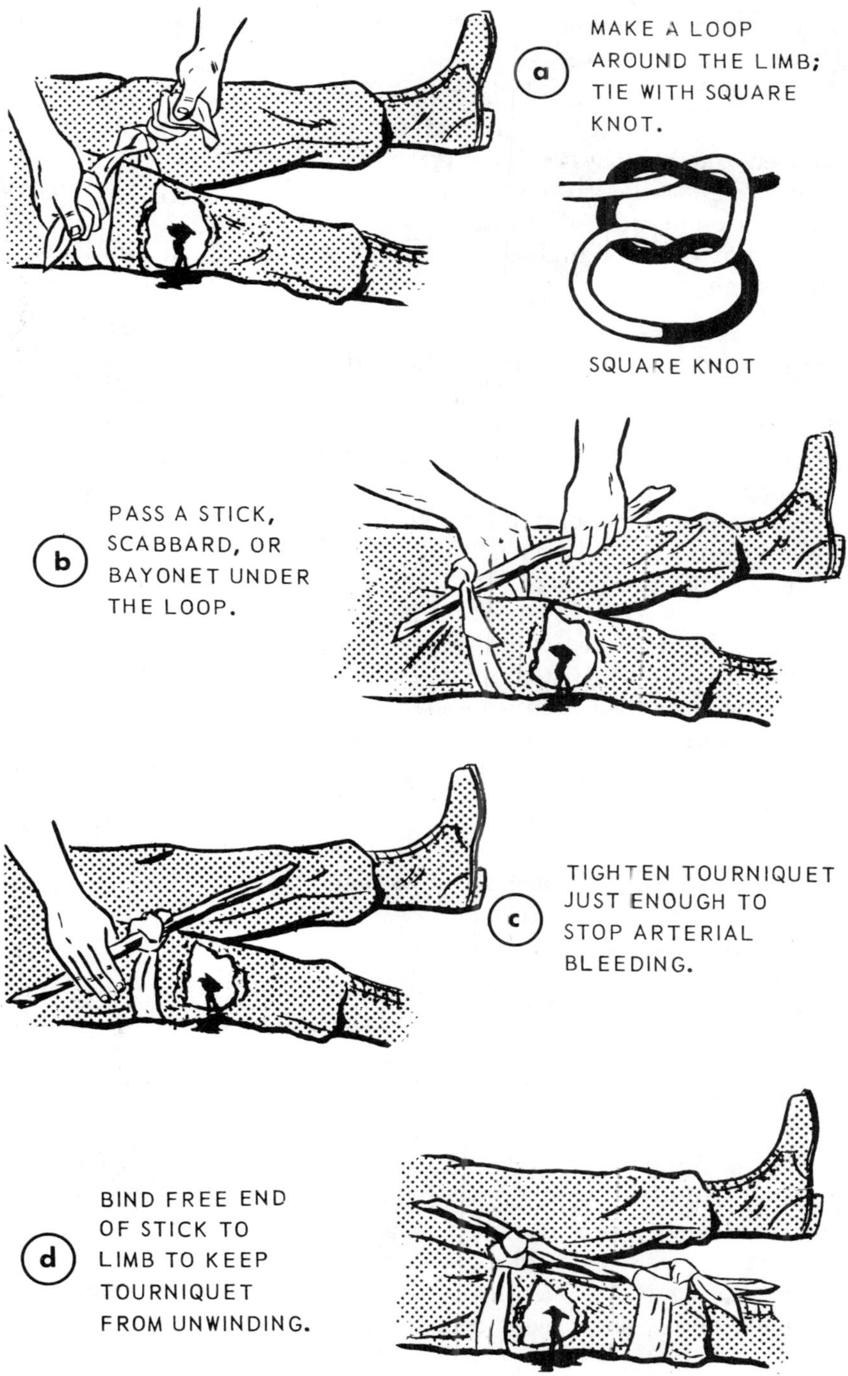

Figure 16. Application of an improvised tourniquet.

associated amputation, place the tourniquet immediately above the knee.

(2) When possible, place the tourniquet over the smoothed sleeve or trouser leg to prevent the skin from being pinched or twisted (fig 15 and 16). Damaging the skin may deprive the surgeon of skin required to cover the amputation stump, thus forcing amputation of more of the limb than might otherwise be necessary. Protection of the skin also reduces the amount of pain inflicted on the casualty.

c. Tightening the Tourniquet. Tighten the tourniquet is illustrated in figure 15 and 16. Tighten it only enough to stop blood from passing under it. If a pulse can be felt in the intact wrist or foot of the affected limb before the tourniquet is applied, stoppage of this pulse can be used as the indicator that tourniquet pressure is sufficient. To detect a pulse, place two fingers, not the thumb, over the pressure point in the wrist or ankle (fig 14). If such a pulse cannot be used as an indicator, you must rely upon your judgment of reduction of blood flow from the wound. In this case, it will be necessary to uncover the wound temporarily to observe the blood flow. After a tourniquet is properly tightened, arterial (spurting) bleeding will immediately cease; but bleeding from veins (para 4*a*(2) (*b*)) in the lower part of the limb will continue until vessels are drained of the blood already in them. You should NOT continue to tighten the tourniquet in an attempt to stop this drainage.

d. Dressing the Wound. After the tourniquet has been secured in place (fig 15 and 16), dress and bandage the wound as illustrated in figure 13 or as explained in paragraphs 15–18, depending upon the supplies available.

e. Marking the Casualty. If the condition of the casualty or the weather makes it necessary to cover the casualty, leave the tourniquet exposed so that it can be readily seen. If possible, mark the casualty with a "T" on his forehead and indicate the time that the tourniquet was applied.

f. Inspecting the Tourniquet and Dressing. Once a tourniquet has been applied, inspect it and the dressing frequently to see if the tourniquet has slipped and if any sign of further bleeding is present. If necessary, tighten the tourniquet but under no circumstances loosen it. Once a tourniquet has been applied, it must not be loosened by anyone except competent medical personnel.

Section III. LIFESAVING MEASURES C: ADMINISTER SHOCK CONTROL

13. General

a. Shock (para 5*c*) may result from any type of injury. The more severe the injury, the more likely shock is to develop. The early signs of shock are restlessness, thirst, paleness of the skin, and a rapid heartbeat. A casualty in shock may be excited, or he may be calm and appear very tired. He may be sweating even though his skin feels cool and clammy. As shock becomes worse, the casualty breathes in small, fast breaths or gasps even when his airway is clear. He may stare vacantly into space. His skin may have a blotchy or bluish appearance, especially around the lips and mouth.

b. Your objective is to administer first-aid measures which will prevent shock from developing or getting worse. All of the measures discussed in paragraph 14 help to prevent or control shock.

14. Shock Control Measures

a. Maintain Adequate Respiration and Heartbeat. To maintain adequate respiration and heartbeat, you may need to do nothing more than clear the casualty's upper airway (para 7), position him to insure adequate drainage of any fluid obstructing his airway (*f* below), and observe him to insure that his airway remains unobstructed. You may need to administer artificial respiration and closed-chest heart massage (para 8 and 9).

b. Control Bleeding. Control bleeding application of pressure dressing, by elevation of part, and by use of pressure points as appropriate (para 11*c*(2)). Apply tourniquet if necessary (para 12).

c. Loosen Constrictive Clothing. Loosen clothing at the neck and waist and at other areas in which it tends to bind the casualty. Loosen but do not remove shoes.

d. Reassure the Casualty. Take charge. Show the casualty by your calm self-confidence and gentle yet firm actions that you know what you are doing and that you expect him to feel better because you are helping him. Be attentive but initiate conversation only to give instructions or warnings or to obtain necessary information. If the casualty asks questions regarding the seriousness of his injury, explain that a medical officer will have to examine him in order to determine the extent of injury. Remember, ill-timed or erroneous information can increase the casualty's anxiety.

e. Splint Fractures. If the casualty has a fracture, splint the part as described in chapter 3.

f. Position the Casualty. The position in which the casualty should be placed varies, depending upon the type of wound or injury and whether the casualty is conscious or unconscious. Unless the casualty has an injury for which a special position is prescribed (chap 3), gently place him on a blanket or another suitable protective item (*g* below) in one of the following positions:

(1) If the casualty is conscious, place him on his back on a level surface with his lower extremities elevated 6 to 8 inches to increase the flow of blood to his heart (a, fig 17). This may be accomplished by placing his pack or another suitable object under his feet. Remember, however, do not move a casualty who has a fracture until it has been properly splinted.

(2) If the casualty is unconscious, place him on his side or on his abdomen with his head turned to one side to prevent his choking on vomitus, blood, or other fluid (b, fig 17).

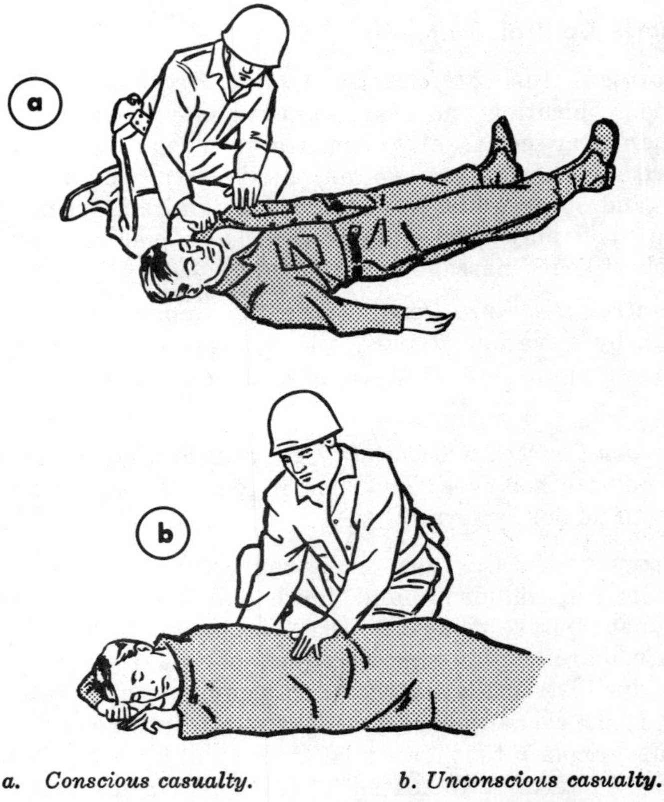

a. Conscious casualty. *b. Unconscious casualty.*

Figure 17. Positioning of a casualty to control shock.

g. Keep the Casualty Comfortably Warm. Do not overheat the casualty. If possible place a blanket, a poncho, a shelter half, or another suitable material under him (*f* above). He may or may not need a blanket over him, depending upon the weather. If the weather permits, remove any wet clothing, except shoes, before covering him.

h. Relieve Pain. Proper dressing and bandaging of wound, splinting of fracture, and positioning of casualty are the best first aid measures for relieving pain.

Section IV. LIFESAVING MEASURES D: APPLY DRESSING AND BANDAGE

15. General

All wounds, except those made under special conditions such as in the operating room, are considered to be contaminated, as infection producing germs are always present on the skin, on the clothing, and in the air. Furthermore, any missile or instrument causing the wound pushes or carries germs into it. Infection results from the multiplication and growth of the germs which invade the wound or a break in the skin. The fact that a wound is contaminated, however, does not lessen the importance of protecting it from further contamination. The fewer germs which invade a wound, the less possibility there is of infection and the greater are the casualty's chances for recovery. You must, therefore, dress and bandage a wound as soon as possible to protect it from further contamination as well as to stop the bleeding.

16. Types of Dressings

Dressings are sterile pads or compresses used to cover wounds. They are usually made of gauze or cotton wrapped in gauze. In the field the most widely used dressing is the first aid dressing with attached bandages (fig 13). Other dressings available under certain conditions are gauze compresses of various sizes and small compresses on adhesive strips (fig 18). For the availability of these compresses, see appendix B.

17. Application of Dressings

a. Cut the clothing and lift it away from the wound to avoid further contamination.

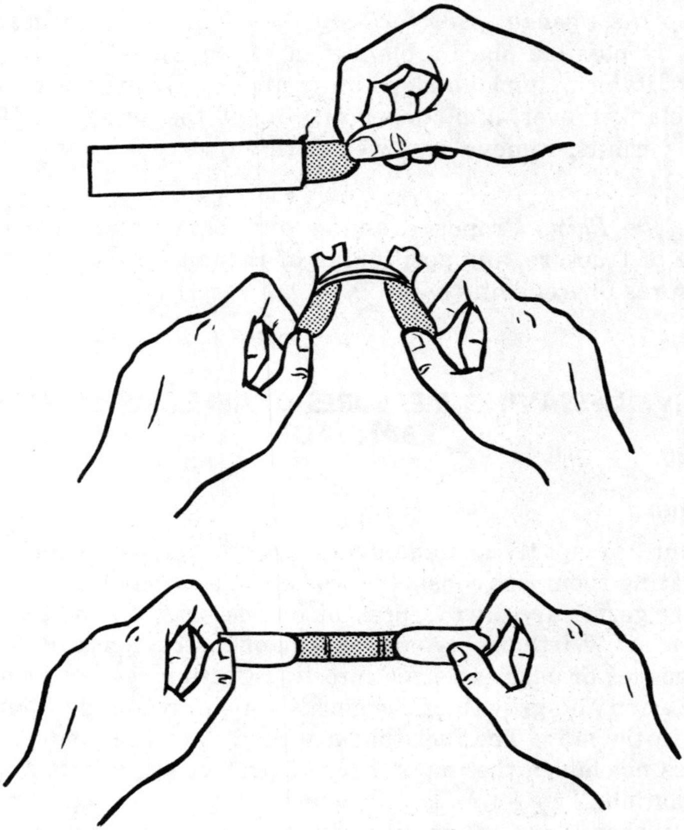

Figure 18. Removal of compress from wrapper.

b. Remove the dressing from its wrapper and place it directly over the wound without letting it touch anything else (fig 13, 18, and 19). For application of dressings to special wounds, see chapter 3.

18. Bandages by Types

A bandage is used over a dressing to hold it in place, to close off its edges from dirt and germs, and to create pressure on the wound for control of bleeding. It is also used to support an injured part or to secure a splint to an injured part (para 30 and 31). A bandage must be applied firmly with the ends secured in place to prevent the bandage and dressing from slipping. A bandage must not be applied so tightly that it stops circulation. If a knot is necessary for securing a bandage, the square knot (fig 15) must be used, as it will not slip. Bandages available to you in the field are made of

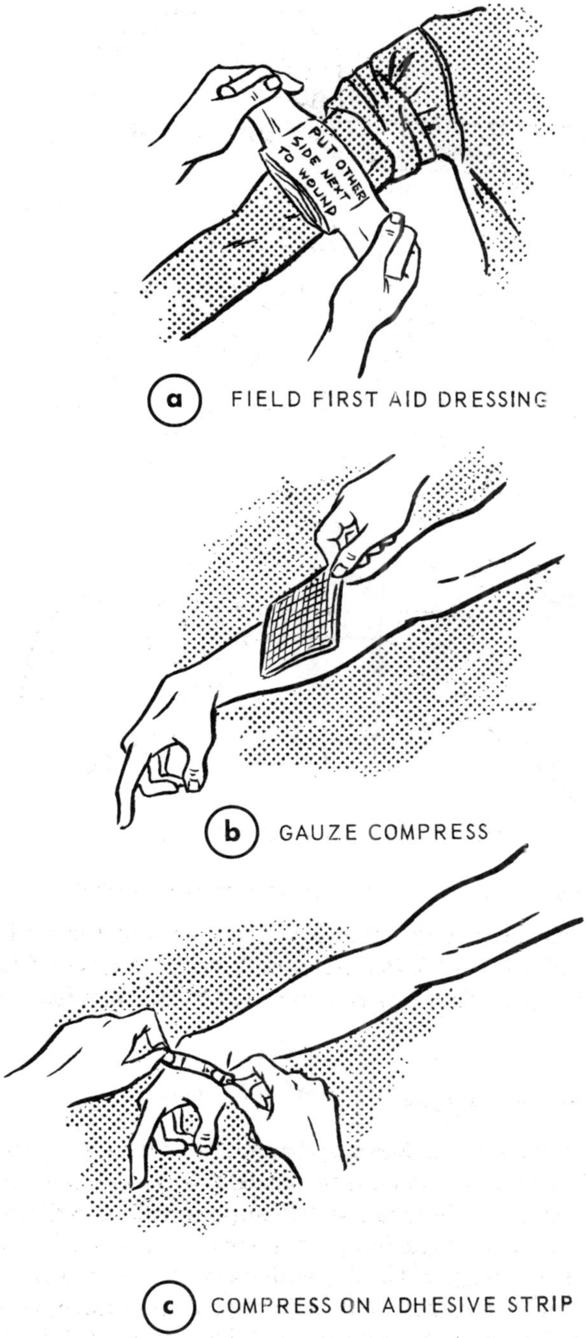

Figure 19. Application of dressings.

either gauze or muslin. The three general types are tailed bandages, triangular and cravat bandages, and roller bandages.

a. Tailed Bandages. Tailed bandages may be attached to the dressing as they are in the field first aid dressing (a, fig 19); or they may be made by splitting a strip of gauze (4 by 36 inches) from each end, leaving the center portion intact to cover the dressing which has been placed over the injured part (fig 20).

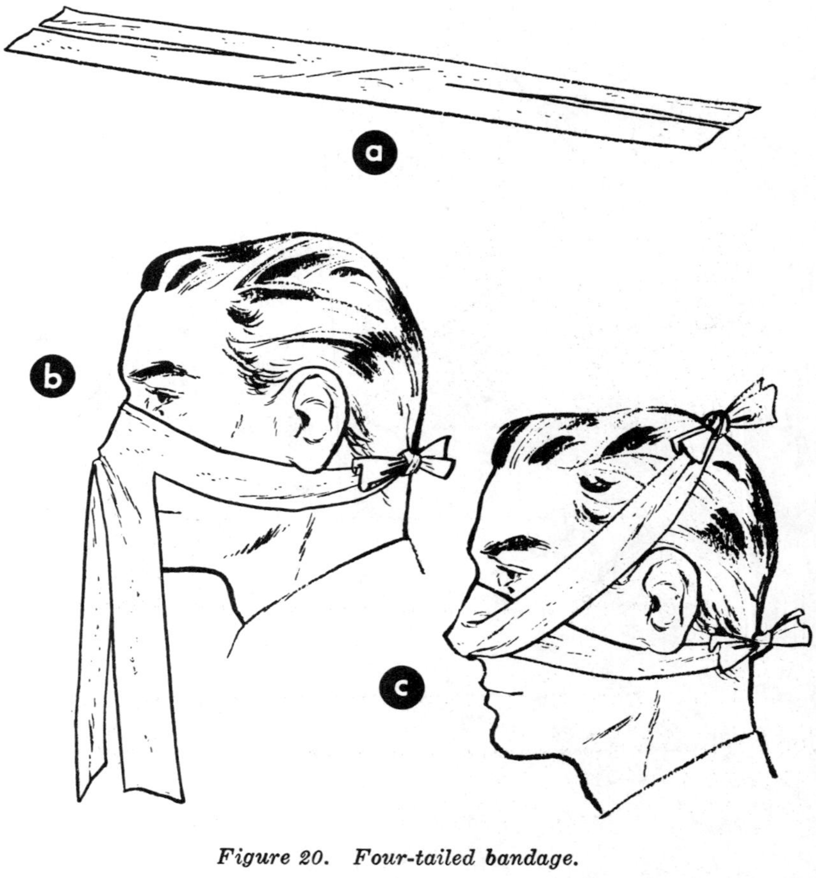

Figure 20. Four-tailed bandage.

b. Trianglar and cravat bandages.

(1) Triangular and cravat bandages are made from the triangular piece of muslin (37 by 37 by 52 inches) provided in the general purpose first aid kit and the Phase I Unit (app B). If this bandage is applied without folding it, it is called a triangular bandage (a, fig 21). If it is folded into a strip, it is called a cravat bandage (b, fig 21). Two safety pins are packed with each bandage.

(2) These bandages are valuable in an emergency, as they are easily applied. They can also be improvised from a piece of shirt, sheet, kerchief, or any other pliable material of a suitable size. To improvise a triangle, cut a square of material somewhat larger than 3 by 3 feet and fold it diagonally. If two bandages are needed, cut the material along the fold.

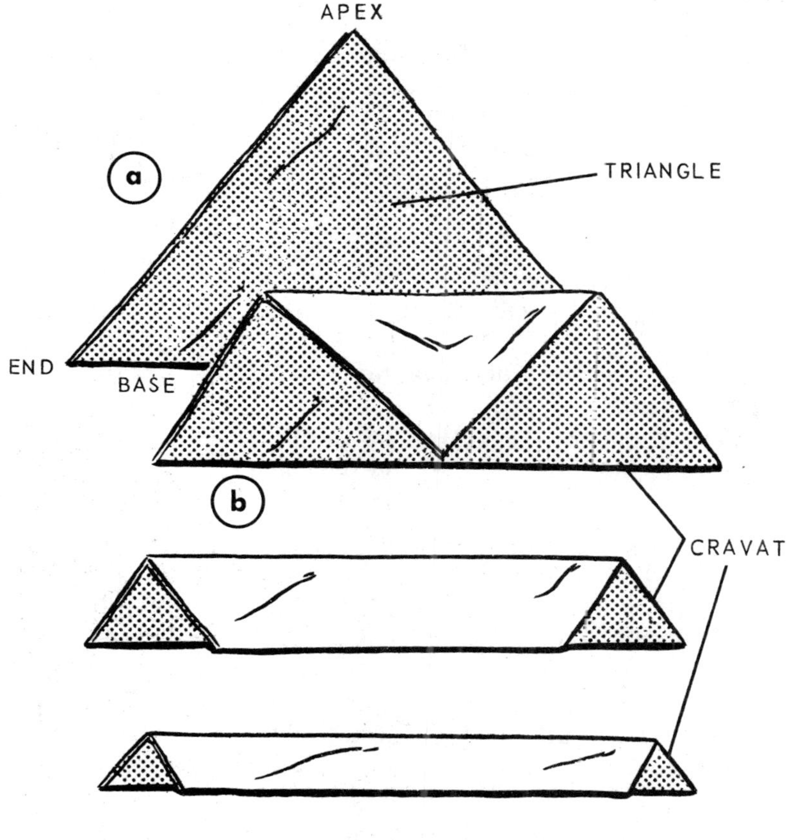

Figure 21. Triangular and cravat bandages.

c. Roller Bandages.

(1) *General.* Roller bandages are made from a roll of gauze (fig 22). The gauze is applied around the injured part in a spiral motion, in a figure-of-eight motion, or in a combination of the spiral and figure-of-eight motions, depending upon the injured part to be bandaged.

(2) *General rules for applying roller bandage.*

(*a*) Apply a roller bandage evenly, firmly, and not too tightly. Excessive or uneven pressure will interfere with circula-

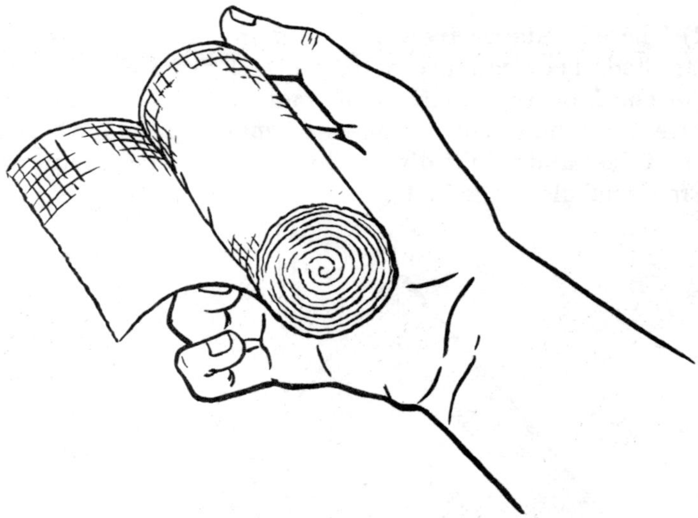

Figure 22. Roller bandage.

tion. At the same time, do not apply it so loosely that it allows the dressing to slip.

(*b*) Bandage the extremity in the position in which you want it to remain, as bending the part after it is bandaged will change the pressure of the bandage.

(*c*) In bandaging an arm or leg, cover the entire extremity (except for the fingers or toes) to maintain uniform pressure. The fingers or toes should be left exposed so the circulation in these parts can be checked.

(*d*) Use a large number of turns rather than a few too firmly applied ones. This is particularly important if the bandage has become wet, such as from a wet dressing. A wet bandage becomes much tighter when it dries; therefore you must allow for shrinkage.

(*e*) Overlap each bandage turn, thus preventing the skin from being pinched between the turns.

(*f*) If two parts are being bandaged together, separate skin surfaces with absorbent material to prevent chafing and irritation.

(*g*) Start the bandaging process by anchoring the bandage securely:

1. Holding the bandage in the right hand with the loose end on the bottom, place the tip of the loose end on the part to be bandaged. Let point of tip extend up (a, fig 23).

2. Using the left hand, bring roll under the part and then over it, transferring the roll back to the right hand.

3. Turn point down (b, fig 23) and extend the bandage

around the part again; thus anchoring the bandage securely (c, fig 23).

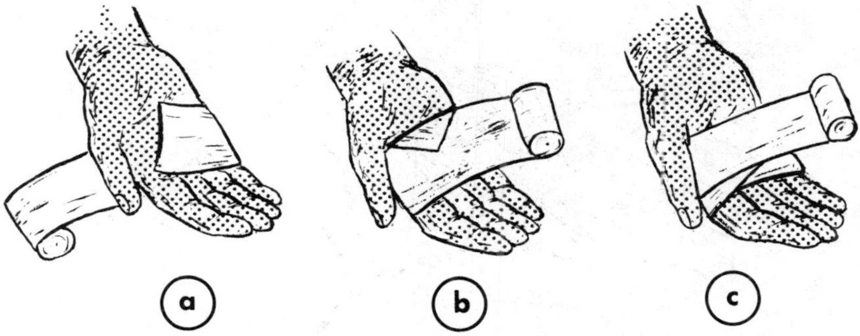

Figure 23. Anchoring the bandage.

(*h*) Bandage the part as appropriate (fig 25 through 58). The dressing (para 16), and any required absorbent material (*f* above) have been omitted in most of the figures in order to illustrate the bandaging technique more clearly.

(*i*) Fasten the bandage securely. To do this, complete the bandaging procedure with several overlying layers of bandage and either pin the loose end to the underlying layers or tie by one of the following methods:

1. Fold the end of the bandage back upon itself and extend it around the part, thus forming two ends; then tie the ends (a, fig 24), using a square knot (fig 15).

2. Split the end of the bandage for a suitable distance; tie a simple knot at the end of the split; extend one end around the part; and tie the two ends (b, fig 24), using a square knot (fig 15).

19. Bandaging of Various Body Parts

a. Head.

(1) *Application of bandages attached to field first aid dressing (a, fig 25).*

(*a*) Cross bandages No. 1 and 2 under chin and tie them on top of head (b, fig 25).

(*b*) Bring bandages No. 4 under chin to meet No. 3 at a point above ear and secure to other bandages (c, fig 25).

(*c*) Take bandages No. 3 and 4 in opposite directions to other side of head and tie them above ear to other bandages with square knot (d, fig 25).

(2) *Triangular bandage (fig 21) applied to head.*

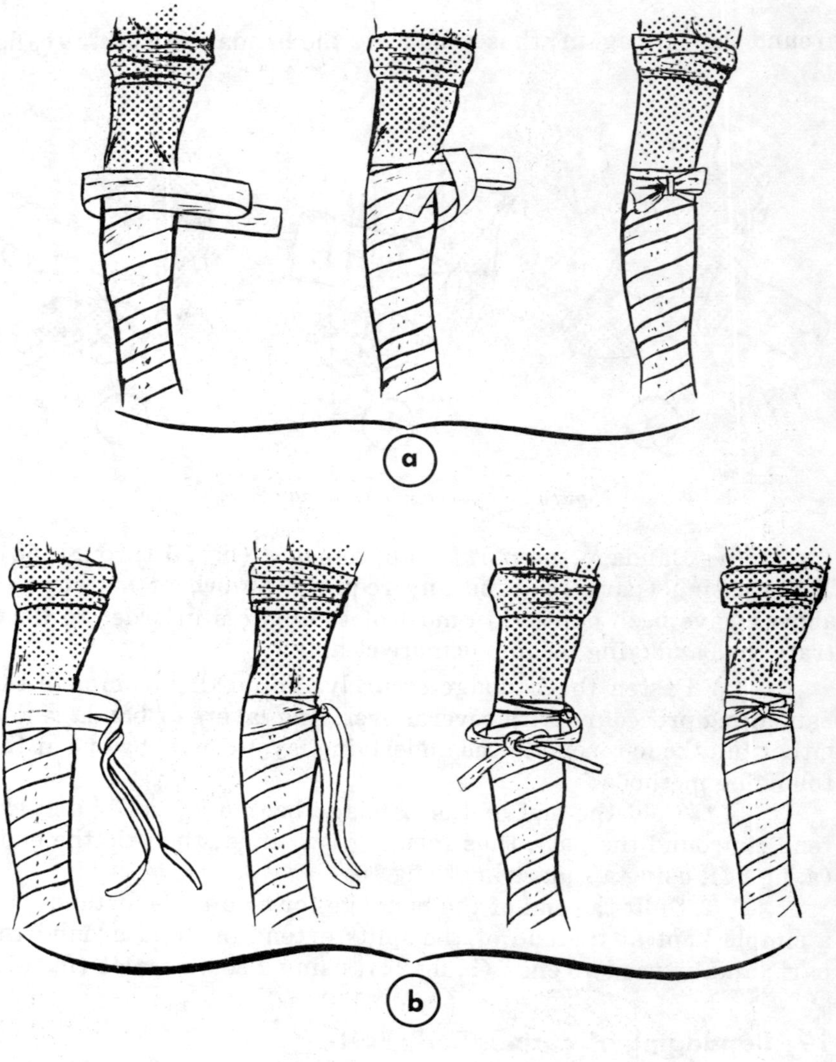

Figure 24. Tying the bandage.

(*a*) Turn base of bandage up and place center of base on center of forehead, letting apex fall on back of neck; then take ends backwards (a, fig 26).

(*b*) Cross ends over apex; then take them over forehead and tie with square knot (b, fig 26).

(*c*) Tuck apex behind crossed part of bandage and further secure it with safety pin, if available (c, fig 26).

(3) *Cravat bandage (fig 21) applied to head.*

(*a*) Place middle portion of bandage over dressing (a, fig 27).

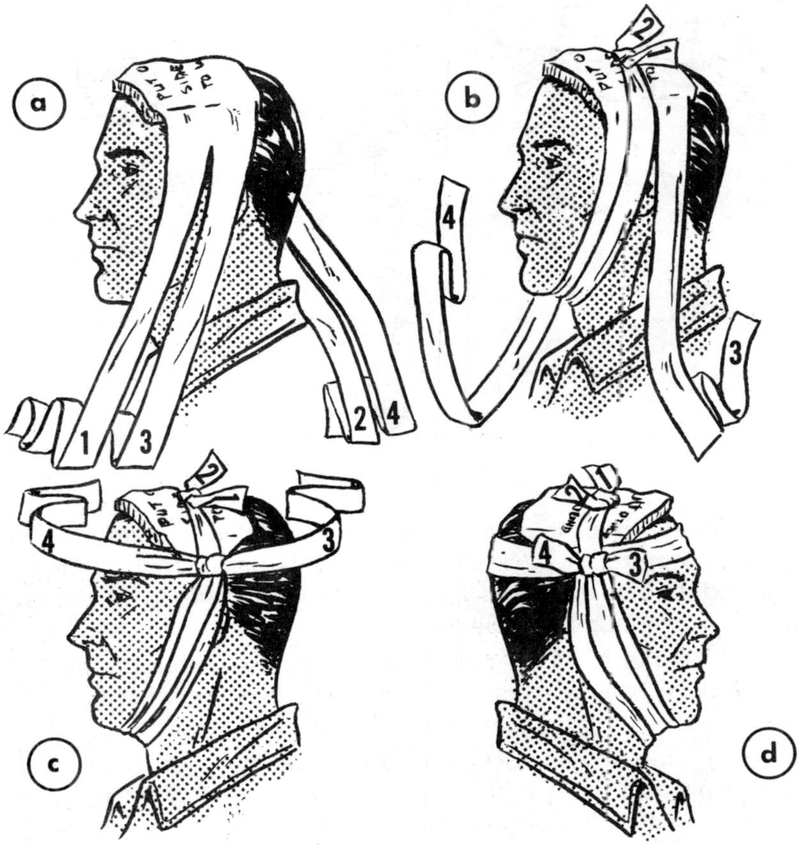

Figure 25. Securing field first aid dressing to head with attached bandages.

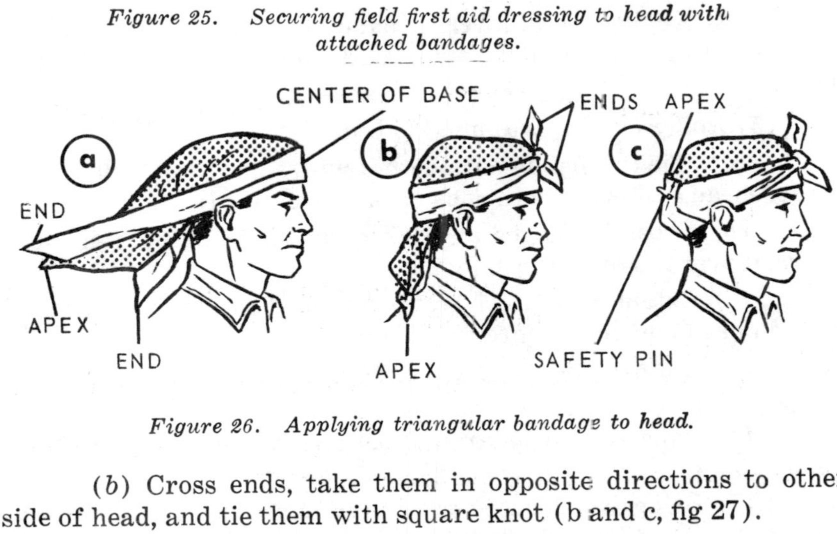

Figure 26. Applying triangular bandage to head.

(*b*) Cross ends, take them in opposite directions to other side of head, and tie them with square knot (b and c, fig 27).

(4) *Roller bandage (fig 22) applied to head.*

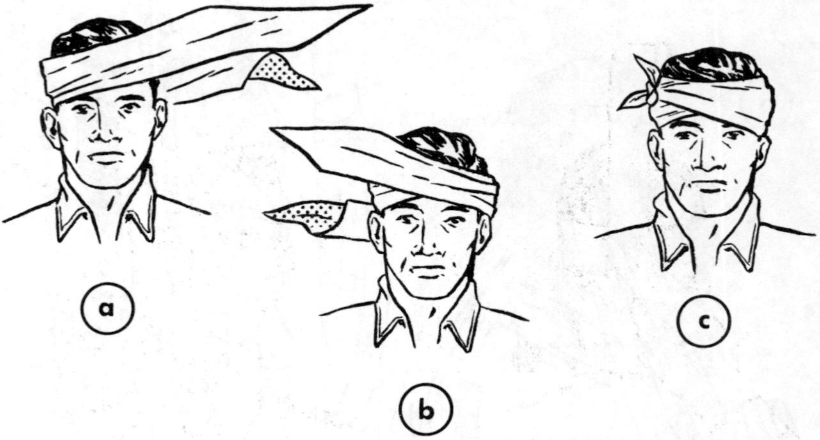

Figure 27. Applying cravat bandage to head.

(*a*) Anchor bandage with several turns around the head (fig 23), stopping at back of head. At this point, fold bandage so that it extends upward and have assistant to casualty hold fold in place with two fingers (a, fig 28).

(*b*) Take bandage over top of head to center of forehead. Fold bandage back at this point and hold it there with free hand (b, fig 28).

(*c*) Take bandage over head to point held by assistant and continue process until entire head is covered, alternating to left and right of middle line and overlapping outer half of preceding layer of bandage (c, fig 28).

(*d*) Apply several layers around head, covering edges; then secure end by pinning or by tying with square knot (fig 24 and d, fig 28).

(5) *Roller bandages applied to head without assistance.*

(*a*) Tie two bandages together with square knot. Place knot on forehead and bring both rolls back above ears (a, fig 29).

(*b*) Cross bandages at back of head, bringing roll No. 1 upward over top of head (b, fig 29).

(*c*) Extend roll No. 1 below forehead and bring roll No. 2 around head and across forehead over No. 1 (c, fig 29).

(*d*) Return roll No. 1 over top of head to back of head (d, fig 29).

(*e*) Take roll No. 2 around back of head and across No. 1 (e, fig 29).

(*f*) Bring No. 1 over top of head again and repeat process until entire head is covered, alternating to left and right of middle

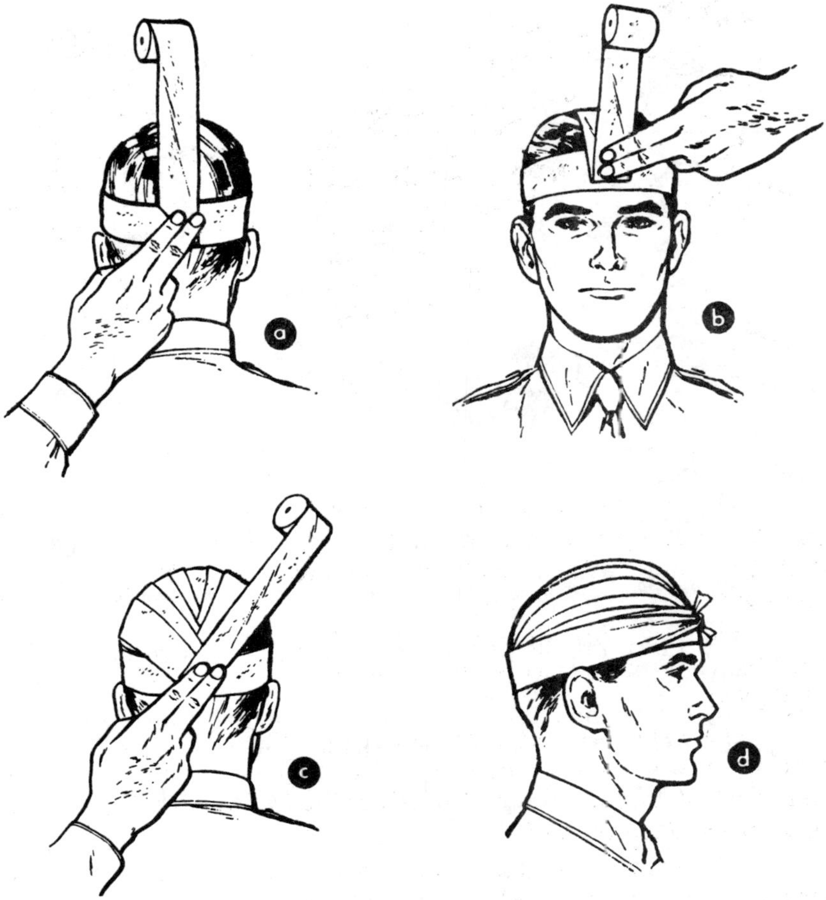

Figure 28. Applying roller bandage to head.

line and overlapping outer half of preceding layer of bandage.

(*g*) Apply several layers around head, securing all edges; then tie ends with square knot (f and g, fig 29).

b. Eye and Ear.

Note. For very minimal injuries, bandaging only one eye may suffice. For any major injury, or in case of any doubt, both eyes must be bandaged. If only one eye is bandaged, the casualty will use his unaffected eye. Since eye movements are synchronized, use of the unaffected eye may result in movement of the affected one, thereby subjecting it to further injury. Also, an eye may have to be bandaged in order to bandage an injury in the area near the eye but not including the eye itself.

(1) *Cravat bandage* (*fig 21*) *applied to eye or ear area* (*fig 30*).

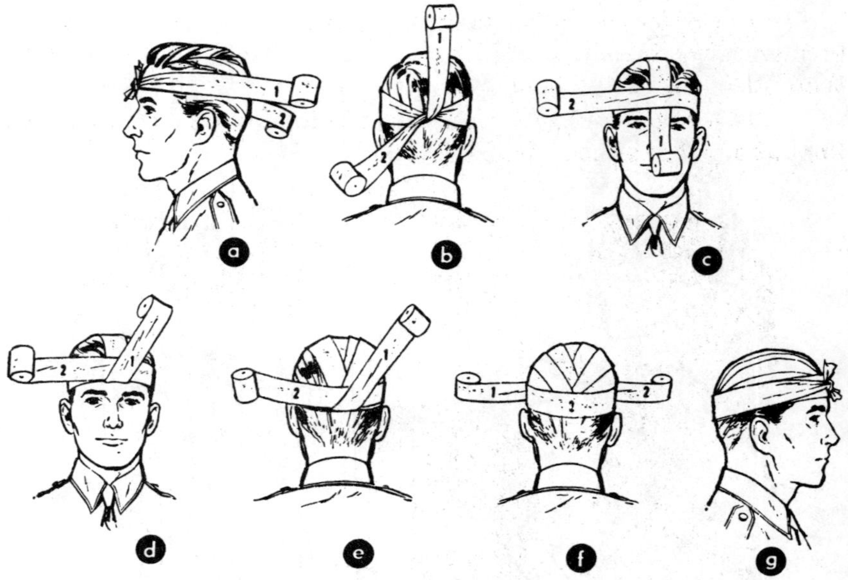

Figure 29. Applying roller bandage to head, using two rolls.

(*a*) Place middle portion of bandage over eye or ear area (a, fig 30).

(*b*) Cross ends, take them in opposite directions around the head, and tie them with square knot (b and c, fig 30).

(2) *Application of cravat bandage (fig 21) to both eyes (fig 31).*

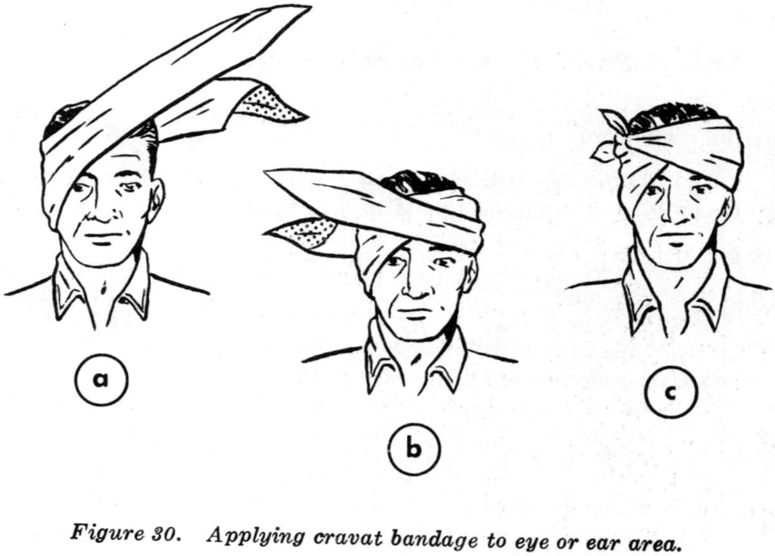

Figure 30. Applying cravat bandage to eye or ear area.

(*a*) Place cravat bandage over eyes, which have been covered with eye dressings, adjusting bandage to make one end longer than other one (a and b, fig 31).

(*b*) Take bandage around head twice and tie ends in square knot at one side of head (c, fig 31).

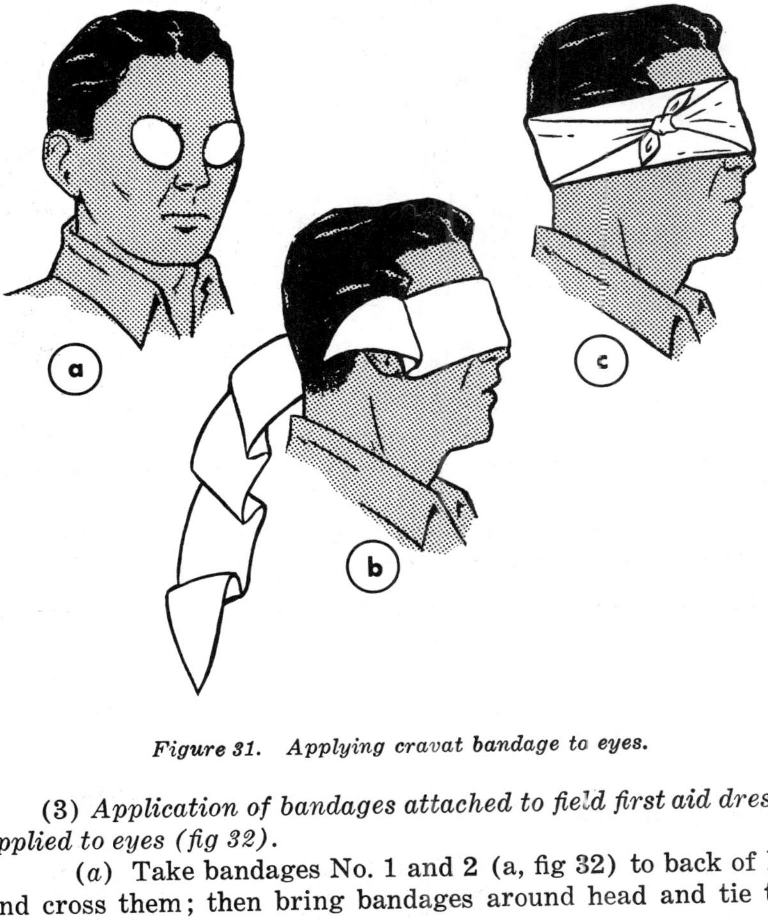

Figure 31. Applying cravat bandage to eyes.

(3) *Application of bandages attached to field first aid dressing applied to eyes (fig 32).*

(*a*) Take bandages No. 1 and 2 (a, fig 32) to back of head and cross them; then bring bandages around head and tie them with square knot (b, fig 32).

(*b*) Cross bandages No. 3 and 4 on top of head and bring longest bandage under chin; then secure bandages No. 3 and 4 to other bandages, and tie them with square knot (c, fig 32).

(4) *Roller bandage (fig 22) applied to eyes.*

(*a*) Anchor bandage with several turns around the head (fig 23 and a, fig 33), stopping at the back of the head.

(*b*) Bring bandage under ear and over one eye to bridge of nose, joining the bandage placed around head (b, fig 33).

(*c*) Take bandage around head, over other eye (c, fig 33),

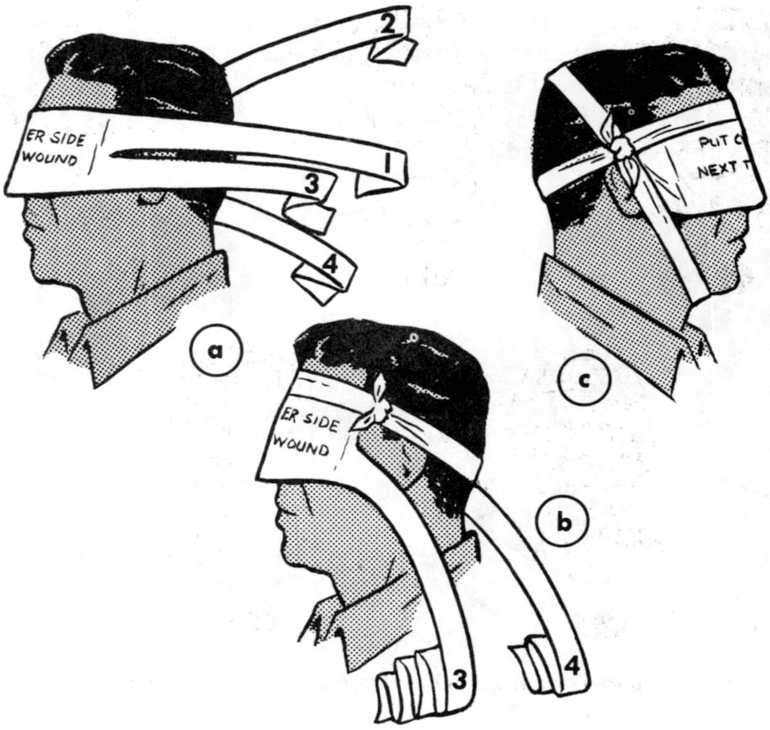

Figure 32. Securing field first aid dressing to eyes with attached bandages.

under ear, and up back of head, joining the bandage placed around head; then take bandage completely around head to secure it.

(*d*) Take bandage to back of head and repeat process, overlapping preceding layer somewhat until eyes are covered (d, fig 33).

(*e*) Secure bandage by applying several layers around head and by pinning end or tying with square knot (fig 24 and e, fig 33).

c. Jaw.

Note. Before applying bandage to a casualty's jaw, take any removable dentures (full or partial) from his mouth and put them in his pocket. In applying the bandage, allow his jaw enough freedom to permit passage of air and drainage from his mouth. To avoid bandaging his mouth completely closed, place a wad of material with a thickness of approximately one-eighth inch between his teeth and gums. To insure that this wad of material does not fall into his mouth and block his airway, leave a streamer of the material attached to the wad and tie it to the bandage.

(1) *Application of bandages attached to field first aid dressing (a, fig 19).* After placing the dressing over the wound, apply the bandages, using the same technique illustrated in figure 25.

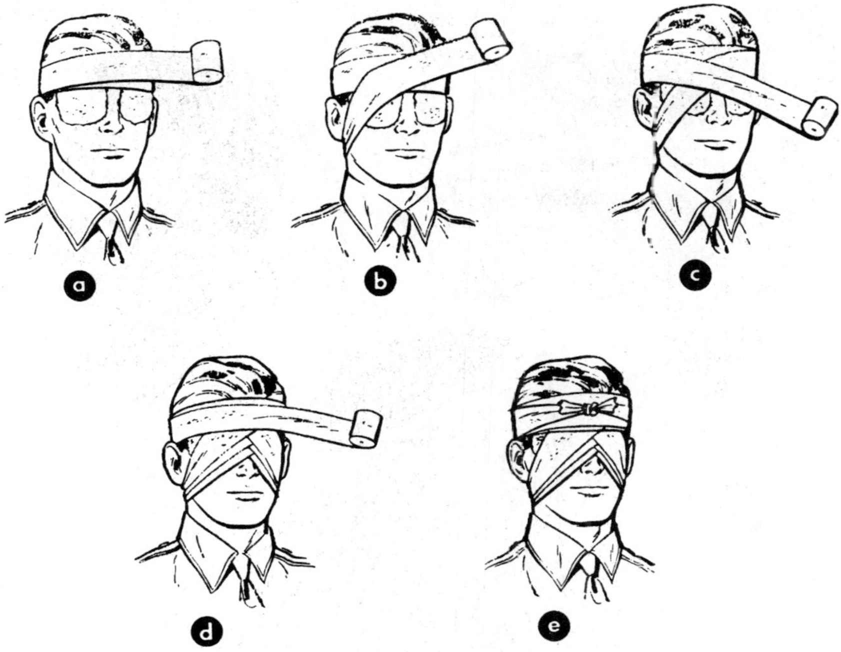

Figure 33. Applying roller bandages to both eyes.

(2) *Tailed bandage (fig 20) applied to jaw.*

(*a*) Place middle portion of bandage over chin; then carry the two upper tails along each side of jaw and tie them with square knot at back of neck (a, fig 34).

(*b*) Turn the middle portion under the chin; then carry the bottom tails in front of ears and tie them with square knot on top of head (b, fig 34).

(3) *Cravat bandage (fig 21) applied to jaw.*

(*a*) Place bandage under chin and carry ends upward; adjust bandage to make one end longer than other one (a, fig 35).

(*b*) Take longer end over top of head to meet short end at temple; then cross ends (b, fig 35).

(*c*) Take ends in opposite directions to other side of head and tie them with square knot over portion applied first (c, fig 35).

(4) *Roller bandage (fig 22) applied to jaw.*

(*a*) Beginning at temple, anchor bandage (fig 23) and take it over head and under chin for several turns as needed; then fold bandage back on finger of other hand and take it around head several times to secure vertical bandage (a, fig 36).

(*b*) Cut bandage and secure end with safety pin (b, fig 36).

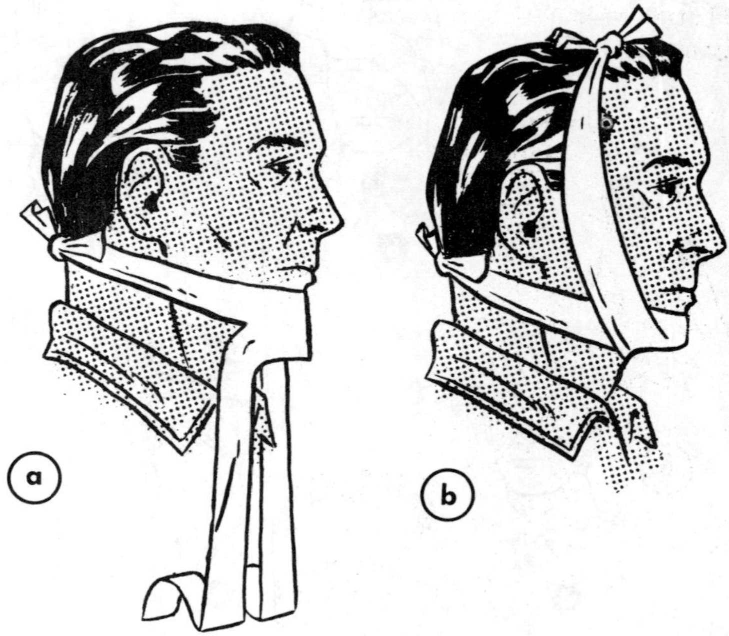

Figure 34. Applying tailed bandage to jaw.

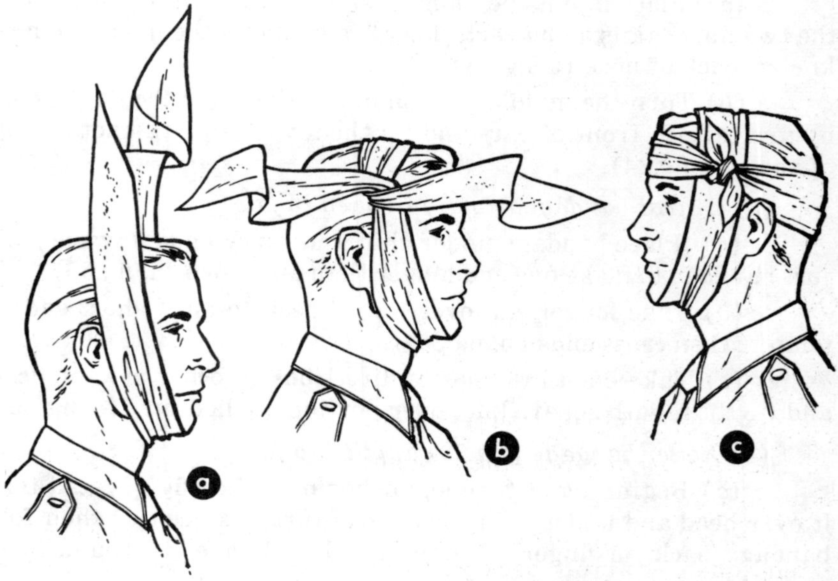

Figure 35. Applying cravat bandage to jaw.

(*c*) To prevent bandage under jaw from slipping, place a folded strip of bandage across chin and secure it on each side with safety pin (c, fig 36).

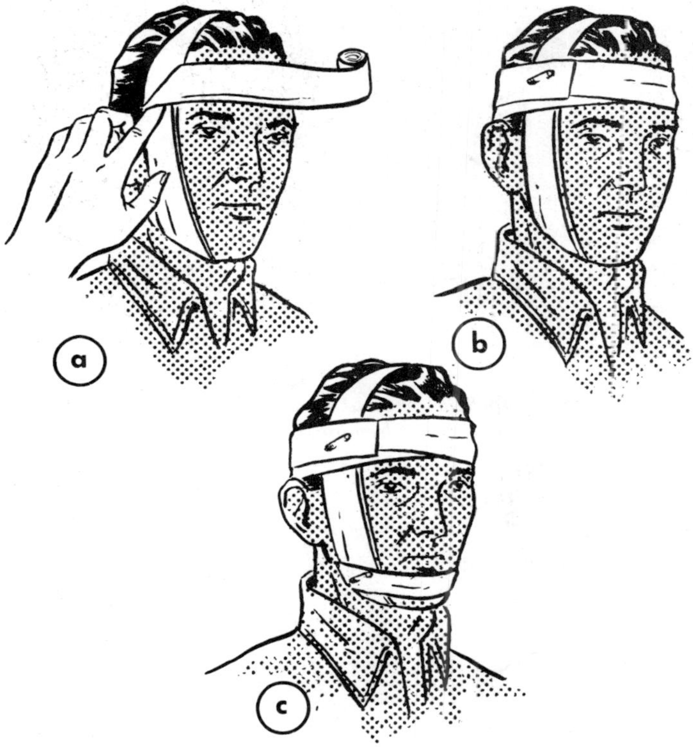

Figure 36. Applying roller bandage to jaw.

d. Shoulder.

(1) *Application of bandages attached to field first aid dressing (fig 37).*

(*a*) Take one bandage across chest and the other one across back and under arm opposite to injured shoulder.

(*b*) Tie ends with square knot.

(2) *Triangular and cravat bandages (fig 21) applied to shoulder.*

(*a*) Place middle of cravat at base of neck on injured side; extend one end across back and under arm and other end across chest; tie ends with square knot (a, fig 38). If necessary, use casualty's belt as a substitute.

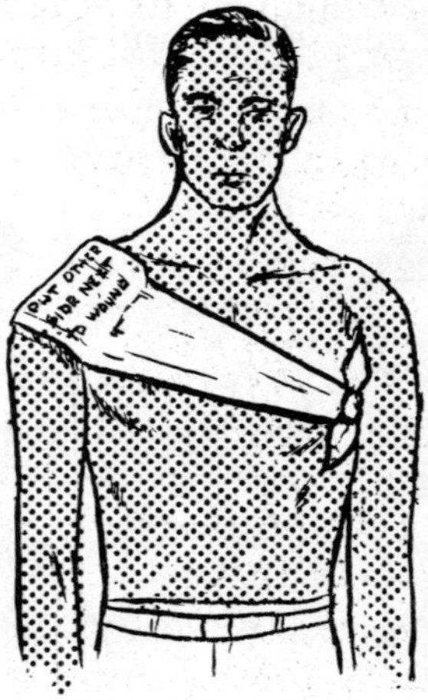

Figure 37. Securing field first aid dressing to shoulder with attached bandages.

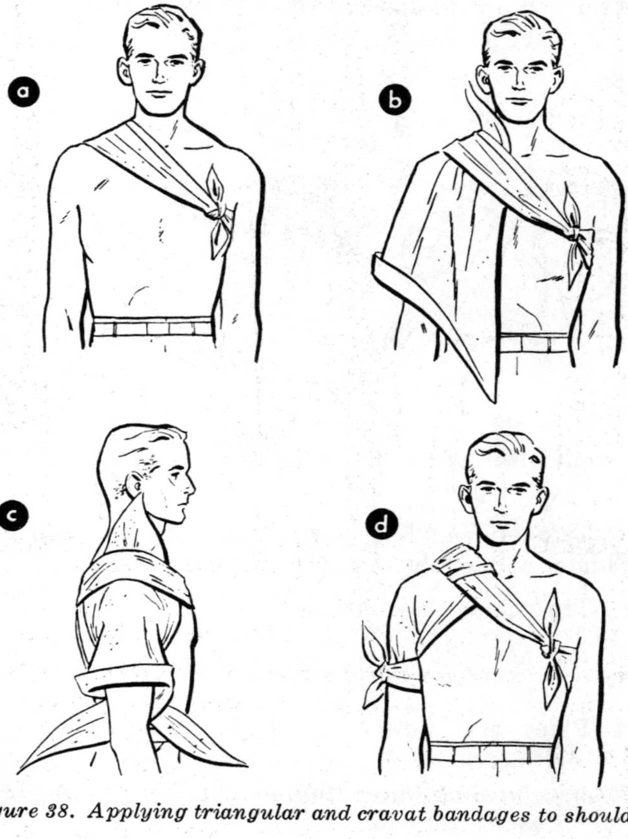

Figure 38. Applying triangular and cravat bandages to shoulder.

(*b*) Slide apex of triangular bandage under cravat at base of neck, letting other part fall over injured shoulder (b, fig 38).

(*c*) Turn up cuff at base of triangular bandage; cross ends under upper arm; then bring them around arm in opposite directions and tie with square knot (c, fig 38).

(*d*) Secure apex at neck by bringing it over and tucking it under the cravat. Pin it with a safety pin as necessary.

(3) *Cravat bandage (fig 21) applied to shoulder or armpit.*

(*a*) Extend length of cravat bandage by placing end of one triangular bandage along middle portion of another one, folding the two bandages into a single cravat, and securing the thicker portion with one or more safety pins.

(*b*) Place middle portion of cravat bandage under armpit so front end is longer than back end and safety pins are on the outside (a, fig 39).

(*c*) Cross ends on top of shoulder (b, fig 39).

(*d*) Take one end across back and under arm on opposite side and other end across chest; then tie ends with square knot (c, fig 39).

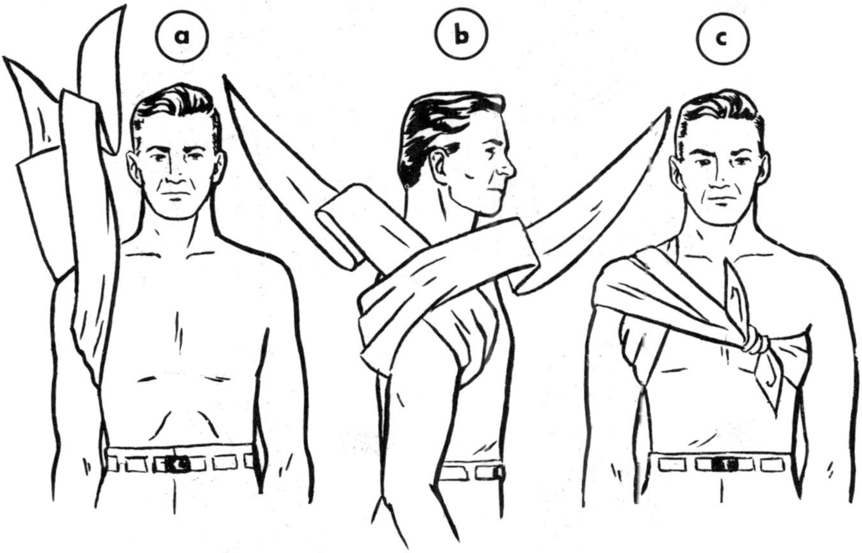

Figure 39. Applying cravat bandage to shoulder or armpit.

e. Chest or Back.

(1) *Triangular and cravat bandages (fig 21) applied to chest or back.*

(*a*) Tie cravat to apex of triangular bandage and place tie to front of shoulder on injured side; then turn base up and place it directly below dressing (a, fig 40).

(*b*) Tie ends of base with square knot on side opposite of injury, leaving one tie longer than other one (b, fig 40).

(*c*) Take cravat bandage over shoulder and tie it to the longer tie of triangular bandage (c, fig 40).

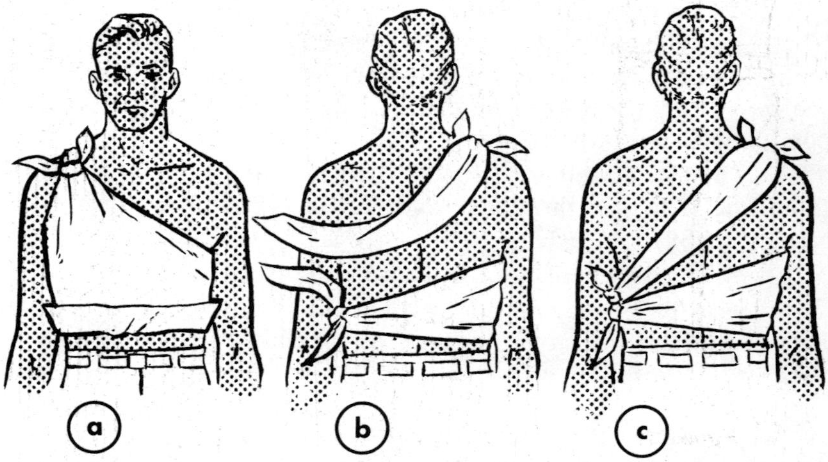

Figure 40. Applying triangular and cravat bandages to chest or back.

(2) Roller bandage (fig 22) applied to chest or back (fig 41).

(*a*) Anchor bandage (fig 23) and apply a number of turns around the body, overlapping preceding layer somewhat.

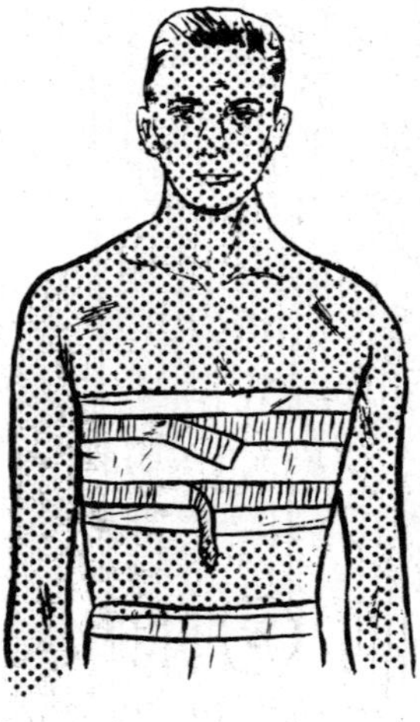

Figure 41. Applying roller bandage to chest or back.

(*b*) Secure the bandage with belts or strips of roller bandage tied with square knot.

f. Hip. Apply triangular and cravat bandages to hip as illustrated in figure 42, using the same techniques described in *d* (2) above to secure the bandages.

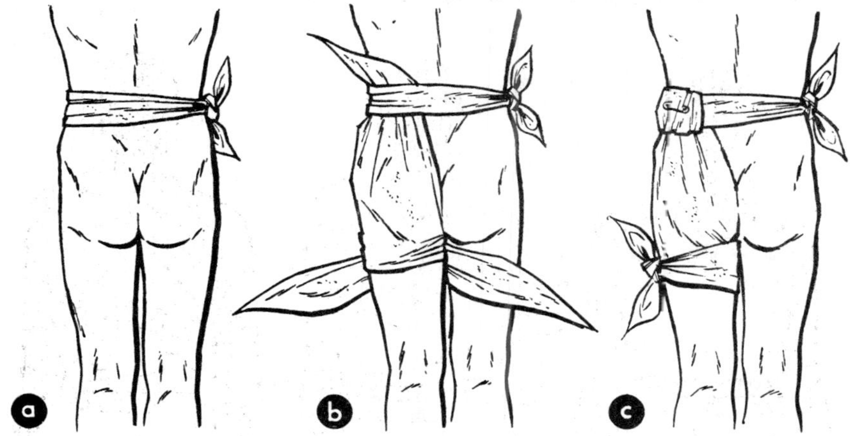

Figure 42. Applying triangular and cravat bandages to hip.

g. Elbow.

(1) *Cravat bandage (fig. 21) applied to elbow.*

(*a*) Bend arm at elbow and place middle of cravat at point of elbow (a, fig 43).

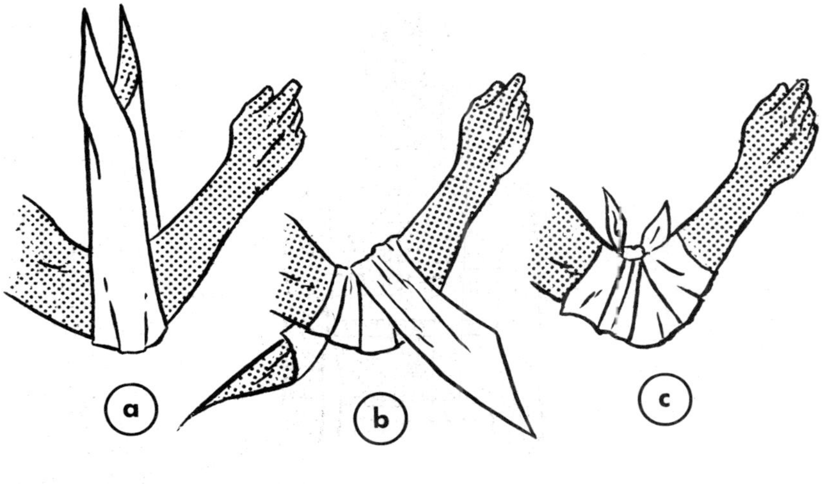

Figure 43. Applying cravat bandage to elbow.

(*b*) Bring ends up and across, extending one downward and one upward (b, fig 43).

(*c*) Take each end around arm and tie with square knot at front of elbow (c, fig 43).

(2) *Roller bandage (fig 22) applied to front of elbow.*

(*a*) Anchor bandage (fig 23) above elbow (fig 44).

(*b*) With arm in a slightly bent position, bring bandage downward and around forearm; then take it upward and around upper arm, thus making a large figure-of-eight motion.

(*c*) Repeat process (*b* above) several times, overlapping each preceding layer somewhat.

(*d*) Secure bandage above elbow by applying several overlying layers and tying with square knot (fig 24).

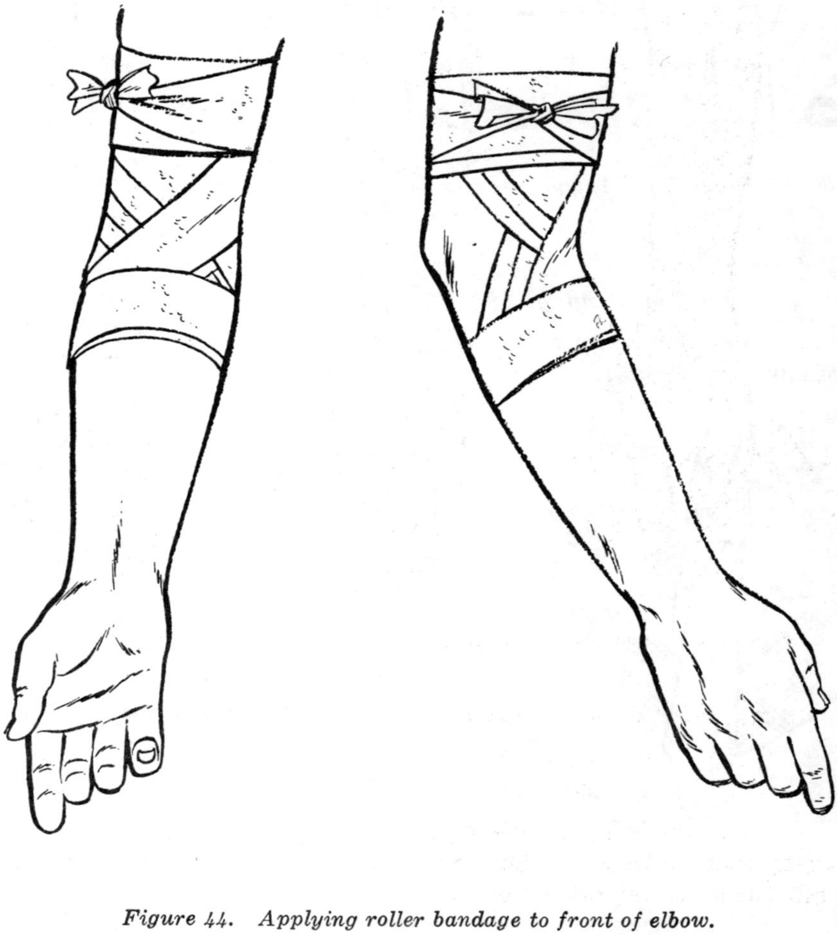

Figure 44. Applying roller bandage to front of elbow.

h. Forearm.

(1) *Roller bandage (fig 22) applied to forearm (spiral technique).*

(*a*) Anchor bandage in palm of hand (fig 23 and a, fig 45).

(*b*) Apply succeeding spiral turns up hand and forearm, overlapping each preceding turn somewhat (b, fig 45).

(*c*) Secure bandage just below elbow by applying several overlying layers and tying with square knot (fig 24 and c, fig 45).

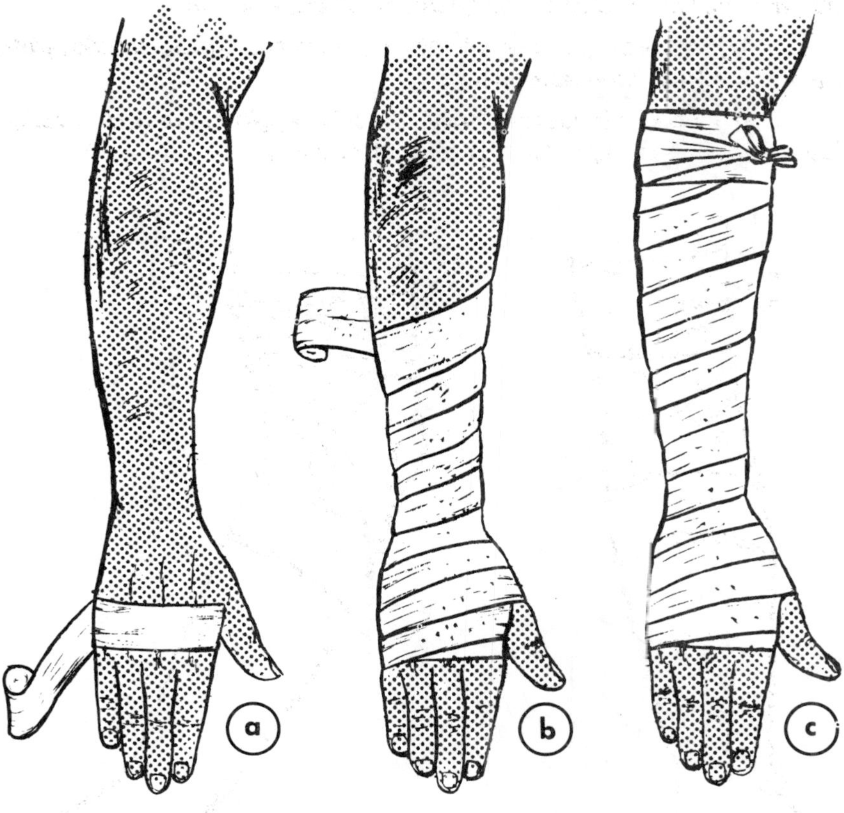

Figure 45. Applying roller bandage to forearm (spiral technique).

(2) *Roller bandage applied to forearm and hand (figure-of-eight technique).*

(*a*) Anchor bandage in palm of hand (fig 23).

(*b*) Apply figure-of-eight turns up the hand and circle the wrist; then extend bandage upward in long spiral motion and circle the arm just below the elbow (a and b, fig 46).

(*c*) Bring bandage downward in long spiral motion and circle the wrist, thus forming an X on the forearm (c, fig 46).

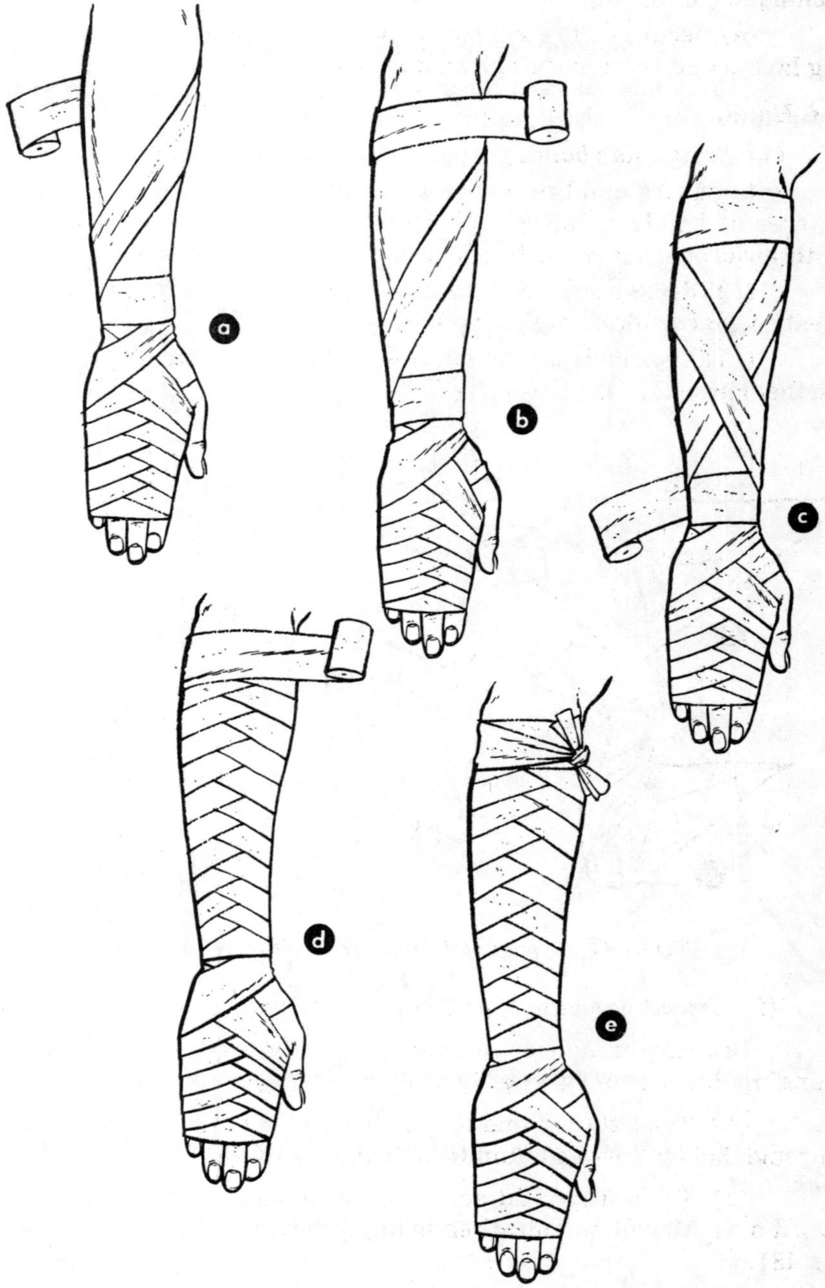

Figure 46. Applying roller bandage to forearm and hand (figure-of-eight technique).

(*d*) Return bandage up forearm, using the figure-of-eight technique (d, fig 46).

(*e*) Secure bandage below elbow by applying several overlying layers and tying with square knot (fig 24 and e, fig 46).

i. Hand.

(1) *Triangular bandage (fig 21) applied to the hand.*

(*a*) Place hand in middle of triangular bandage with wrist at base of bandage (a, fig 47). Insure that fingers are separated with absorbent material to prevent chafing and irritation of skin.

(*b*) Place apex over fingers and tuck excess fullness into pleats on each side of hand (b, fig 47).

(*c*) Cross ends on top of hand, take them around wrist, and tie them in square knot (c–e, fig 47).

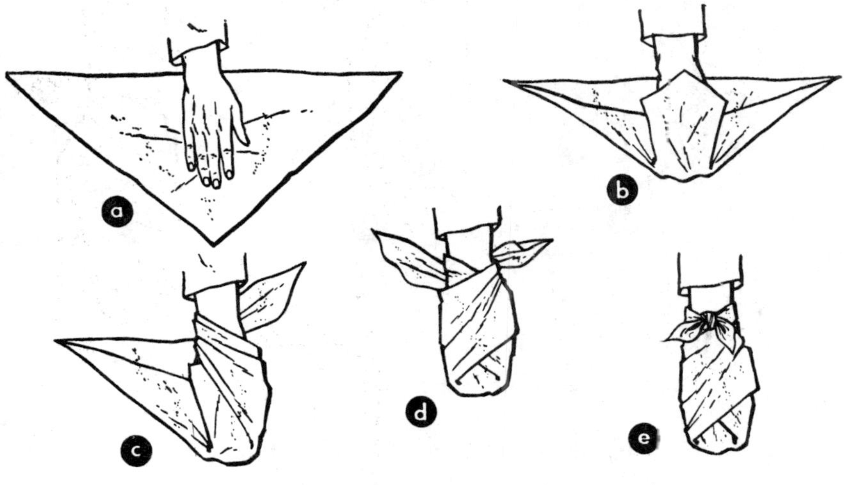

Figure 47. Applying triangular bandage to hand.

(2) *Cravat bandage (fig 21) applied to palm of hand.*

(*a*) Lay middle of cravat over palm of hand with ends hanging down each side (a, fig 48).

(*b*) Take thumb end across back of hand, over palm, and through hollow between thumb and palm (b, fig 48).

(*c*) Take other end across back of hand, extending it upward over base of thumb; then bring it downward across palm (c, fig 48).

(*d*) Take ends to back of hand and cross; then bring them to front of hand and cross again (d and e, fig 48).

(*e*) Tie ends with a square knot at wrist (f, fig 48).

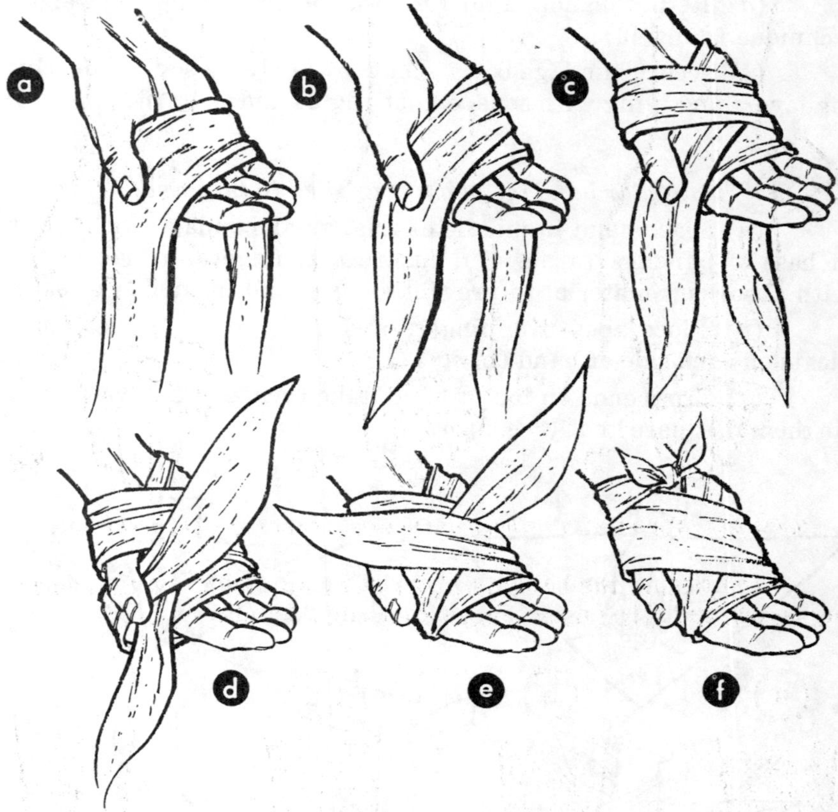

Figure 48. Applying cravat bandage to palm of hand.

(3) *Roller bandage (fig 22) applied to hand.*

(*a*) Anchor bandage (fig 23); then bring it near end of fingers and apply it upward, using the figure-of-eight technique (a, fig 49).

(*b*) At base of fingers, extend the figure-of-eight motion upward to base of the wrist, leaving thumb free (b, fig 49).

(*c*) Secure the bandage at wrist by applying several overlying layers and tying with square knot (fig 24 and c, fig 49).

(4) *Roller bandage applied to back of hand.*

(*a*) Anchor bandage (fig 23) at wrist.

(*b*) Take bandage to back of hand, around base of fifth finger, across back of hand, and around wrist (a, fig 50).

(*c*) Repeat this process with each finger and thumb (b, fig 50).

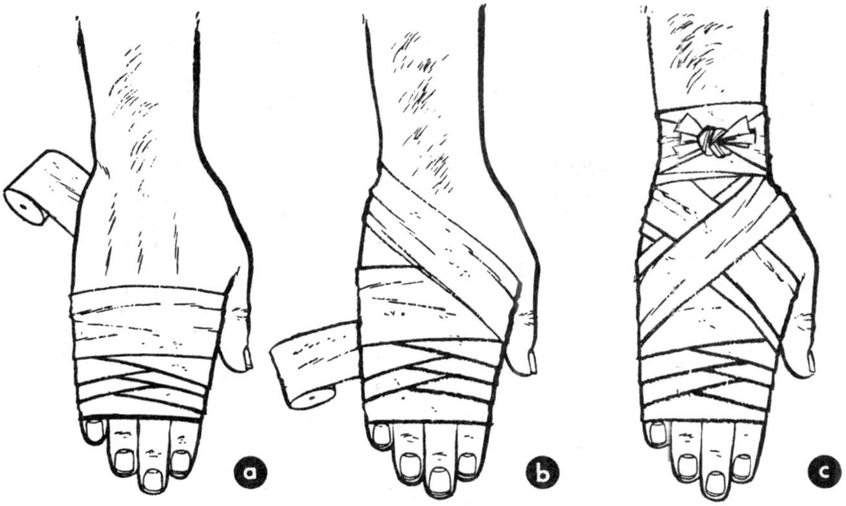

Figure 49. Applying roller bandage to hand (figure-of-eight technique).

(*d*) Secure the bandage at wrist by applying several overlying layers and tying with square knot (fig 24 and c, fig 50).

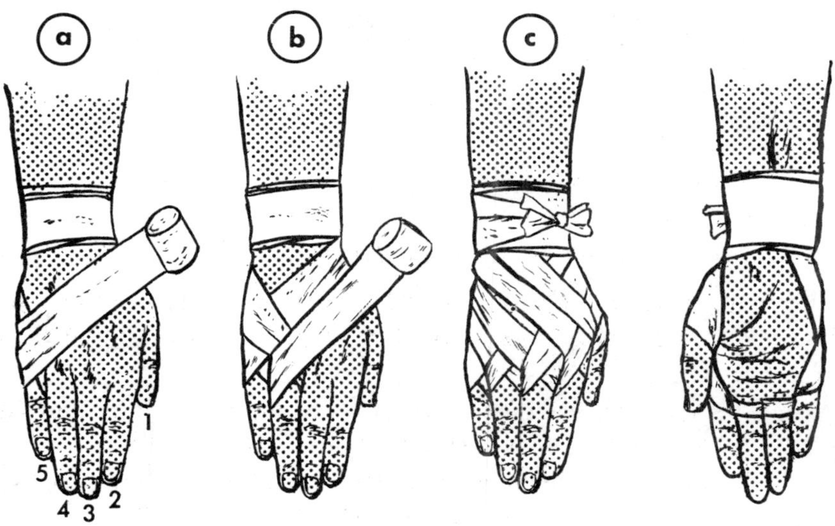

Figure 50. Applying roller bandage to back of hand.

(5) *Roller bandage applied to hand.*

Note. Make certain gauze dressing is placed between fingers (para 18*c* (2)(*f*)).

(*a*) Anchor bandage (fig 23) at wrist.

(*b*) Fold bandage back; then take it over back of hand, under fingers, and up to front of wrist (a, fig 51).

(*c*) Holding folds in place at wrist, continue to take the bandage back and forth until all fingers are covered (b, and c, fig 51).

(*d*) Take bandage around wrist to hold folds in place; then bring bandage across back of hand to tips of fingers and make circular turn. (d and e, fig 51).

(*e*) Apply bandage in a figure-of-eight motion up the hand (f, fig 51).

(*f*) Secure the bandage at wrist by applying several overlying layers and tying with square knot (fig 24 and g, fig 51).

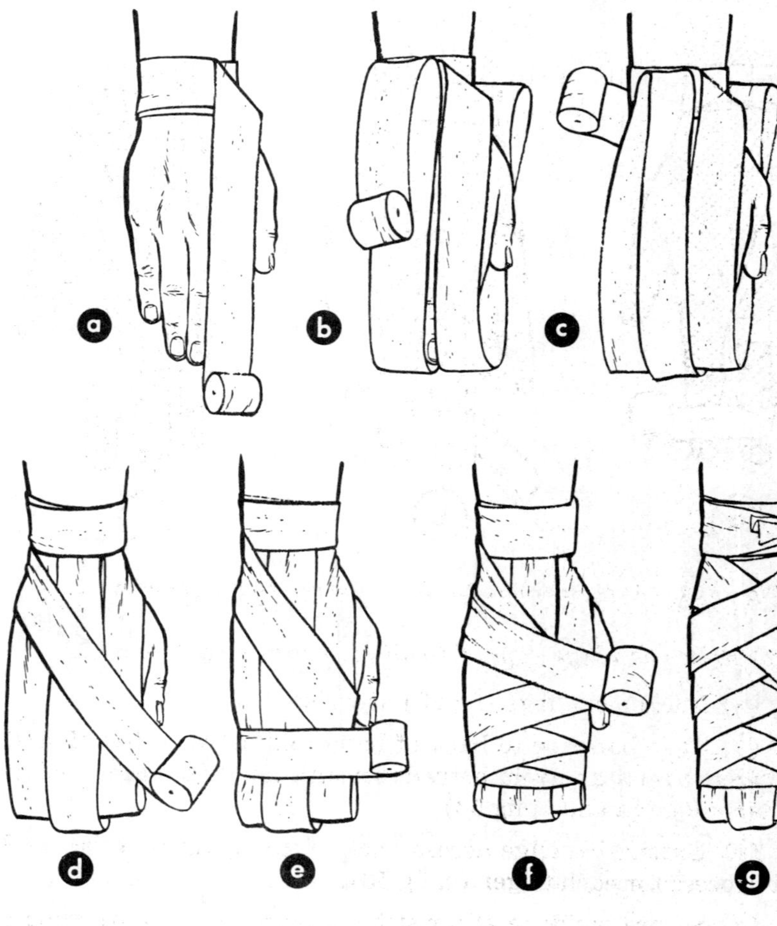

Figure 51. Applying roller bandage to hand.

j. Fingers.

(1) *Roller bandage (fig 22) applied to finger.*

(*a*) Anchor bandage (fig 23) at wrist.

(*b*) Bring bandage over back of hand and make one complete turn at base of injured finger; then take bandage in a long spiral motion to the tip of finger and make one complete turn (a, fig 52).

(*c*) Return the bandage to base and then to tip of finger in long spiral turns (b, fig 52).

(*d*) Apply bandage up finger in small spiral turns and circle finger at its base; then extend bandage across back of hand and secure it at wrist by applying several overlying layers and tying with square knot (fig 24, and c, fig 52).

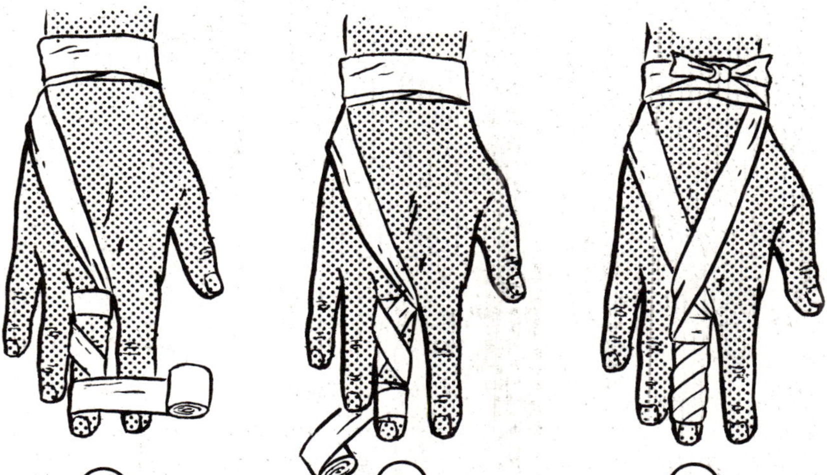

a b c

Figure 52. Applying roller bandage to finger (spiral technique).

(2) *Roller bandage applied to all fingers and back of hand.*

(*a*) Anchor bandage (fig 23) at wrist.

(*b*) Take bandage to back of hand and between fourth and fifth fingers; then apply it both down and up fifth finger, using spiral technique (a and b, fig 53).

(*c*) Extend bandage across back of hand, circle wrist, and repeat process for each finger (c, fig 53).

(*d*) Secure bandage at wrist by applying several overlying layers and tying with square knot (fig 24 and c, fig 53).

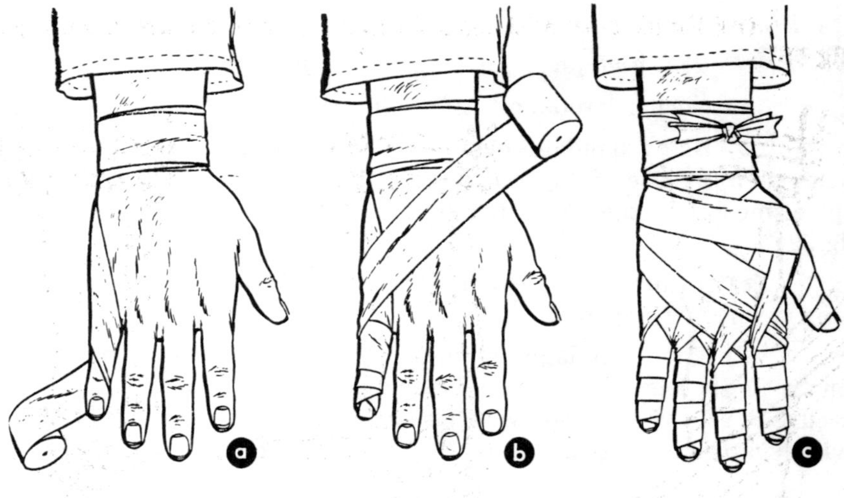

Figure 53. Applying roller bandage to all fingers and back of hand (spiral technique).

k. Knee. Apply cravat bandage to knee as illustrated in figure 54, using the same technique described in *g* (1) above.

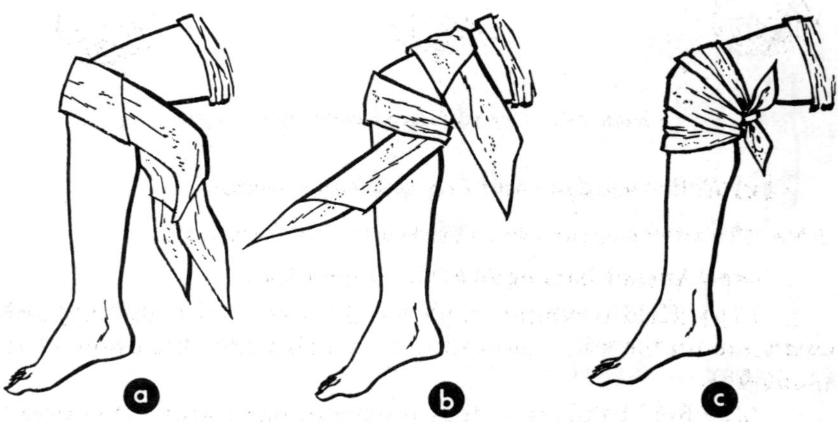

Figure 54. Applying cravat bandage to knee.

l. Leg.

(1) *Cravat bandage (fig 21) applied to the leg.*

(*a*) Place center of cravat over dressing (a, fig 55).

(*b*) Take one end around and up the leg in a spiral motion and the other end around and down the leg in a spiral motion, overlapping part of each preceding turn (b, fig 55).

(*c*) Bring both ends together and tie with square knot (c, fig 55).

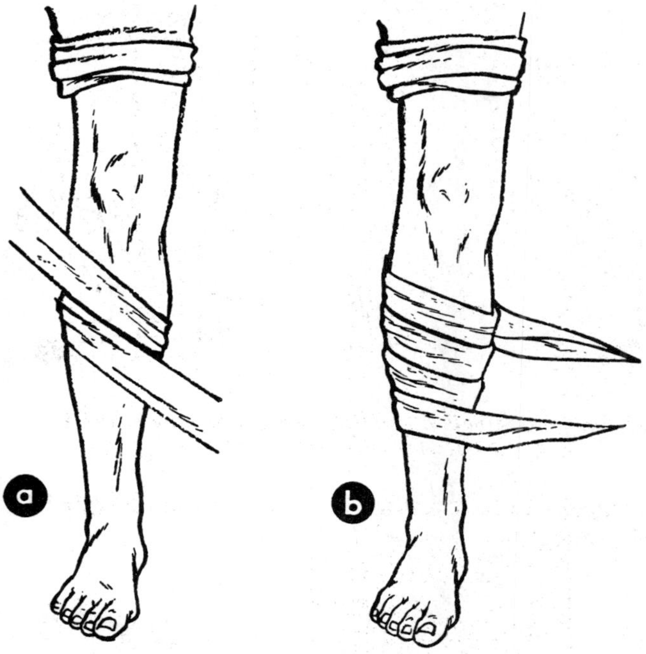

Figure 55. Applying cravat bandage to leg.

(2) *Roller bandage (fig 22) applied to stump.*

Note. This technique can be applied to any extremity.

(*a*) Anchor bandage (fig 23) below knee.

(*b*) Hold dressing in place with loose spiral turn applied down and up the stump and secured with circular turn below knee (a, fig 56).

(*c*) Fold bandage so that it extends downwards; then carry bandage down outer half of stump, over end, and up back of stump to knee (b, fig 56).

(*d*) Holding bandage in place below knee, loop it back and forth as described above to cover inner and middle portion of stump (c, fig 56). It is advisable to apply several additional loops over stump.

(*e*) Secure ends of loops in place by applying several circular turns below knee (d, fig 56).

(*f*) Using a spiral motion, extend bandage to end of stump; then circle stump near end (e, fig 56).

(*g*) Apply bandage up stump, using the figure-of-eight technique (f, fig 56).

(*h*) Secure bandage below knee by applying several overlying layers and tying with square knot (fig 24 and f, fig 56).

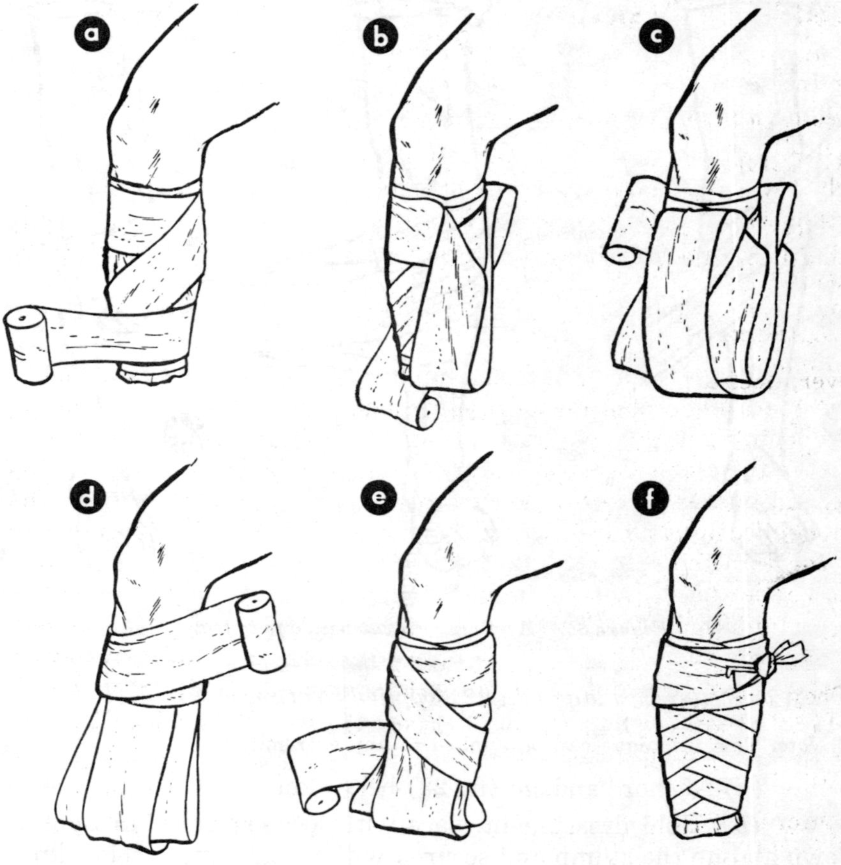

Figure 56. Applying roller bandage to stump.

m. Foot.

(1) *Triangular bandage (fig 21) applied to foot.*

(*a*) Place foot in middle of triangular bandage with heel well forward of base (a, fig 57).

(*b*) Place apex over top of foot and tuck excess fullness into pleats on each side of foot (b, fig 57).

(*c*) Cross ends on top of foot, take them around ankle, and tie them in square knot at front of ankle (c–e, fig 57).

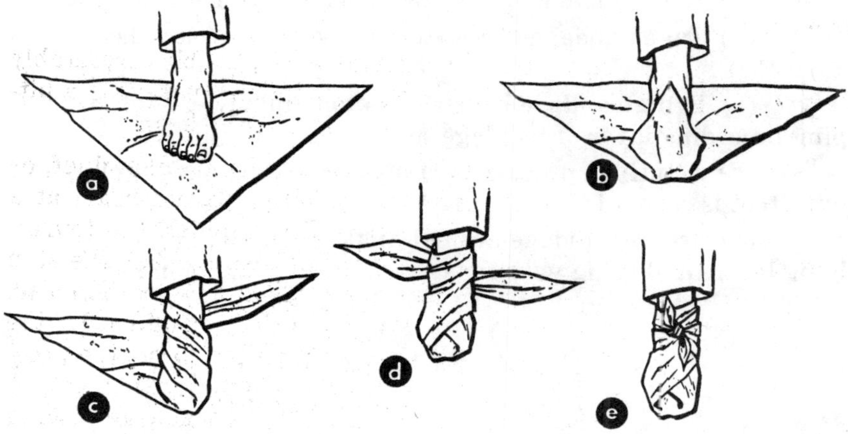

Figure 57. Applying triangular bandage to foot.

(2) *Roller bandage (fig 22) applied to foot.*

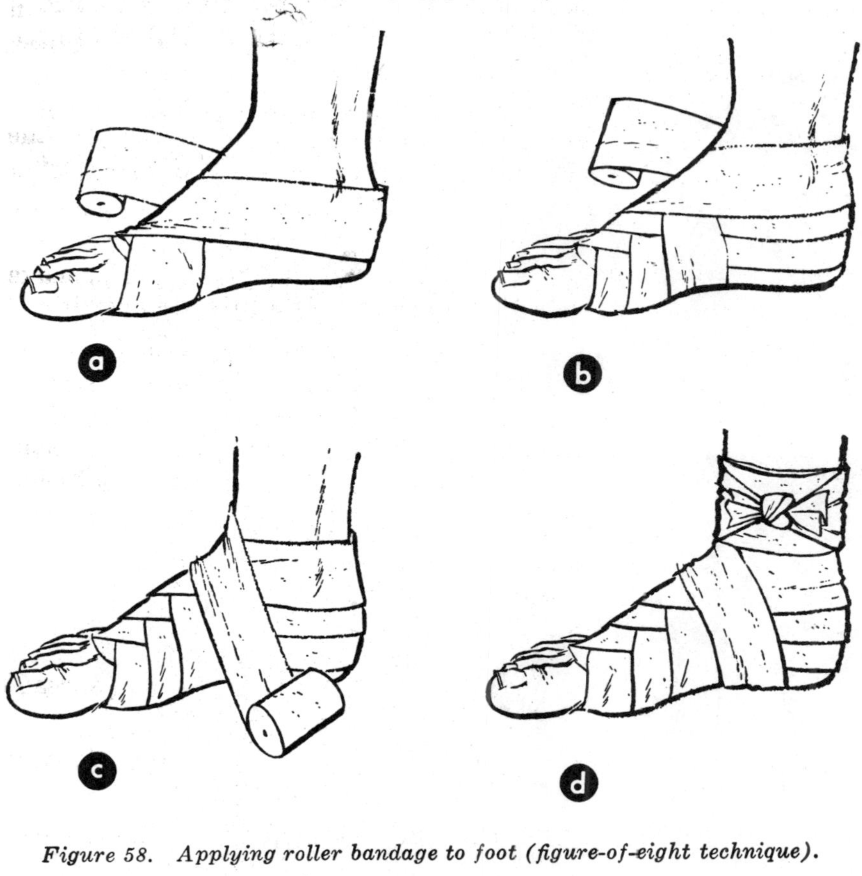

Figure 58. Applying roller bandage to foot (figure-of-eight technique).

(*a*) Anchor bandage (fig 23) around foot near base of toes.

(*b*) Take bandage across top of foot and around heel (a, fig 58).

(*c*) Bring bandage back across top and under foot, overlapping preceding layer of bandage somewhat.

(*d*) Continue process ((*c*) above) in figure-of-eight motion until foot is covered (b and c, fig 58).

(*e*) Secure bandage around ankle by applying several overlying layers and tying with square knot (fig 24 and d, fig 58).

CHAPTER 3

INJURIES REQUIRING SPECIAL FIRST-AID MEASURES

Section I. SEVERE WOUNDS AND BURNS

20. General

The four lifesaving measures discussed in chapter 2 apply to the first aid for all injuries; however certain types of injuries require special precautions and procedures or modifications in the measures previously discussed. These include head injuries, face and neck wounds, sucking wounds of the chest, abdominal wounds, and burns as well as fractures discussed in section II.

21. Head Injuries

a. General. A head injury may consist of one of the following conditions or of a combination of them: a cut or bruise of the scalp; a fracture of the skull with injury to the brain and/or to the blood vessels of the scalp, skull, and brain. Usually, serious skull fractures and brain injuries occur together. A head injury with scalp wound is easily recognized. It is the injury of the head without a scalp wound that will be more difficult for you to recognize. You should, therefore, check for a head injury if the casualty—

(1) Is or has recently been unconscious.

(2) Has blood or other fluid escaping from his nose or ears.

(3) Has a slow pulse (para 4*a*(2)(*a*)).

(4) Has a headache.

(5) Is nauseated or is vomiting.

(6) Has had a convulsion.

(7) Is breathing very slowly.

b. Special Precautions in A B C D Lifesaving Measures (chap 2).

(1) Leave any protruding brain tissue as it is, and apply a sterile dressing over this tissue. Furthermore, do not remove or disturb any foreign matter which may be in the wound.

(2) Do not permit the casualty's head to be in a position lower than the rest of his body.

(3) For proper application of bandages to the head, see paragraph 19*a*.

22. Face and Neck Wounds

a. General. Wounds of the face and neck bleed profusely because of the many blood vessels in these parts. Furthermore, the bleeding is difficult to control.

b. Special Precautions and Modifications to A B C D Lifesaving Measures (chap 2).

(1) First, stop any bleeding which may be causing obstruction of the casualty's upper airway; then clear his airway (para 7). There may be pieces of broken teeth or bone and loose bits of flesh, as well as dentures, in his mouth.

(2) If the casualty is conscious and chooses to sit up, have him lean forward with his head down to permit free drainage from his mouth; otherwise place him in the shock position for an unconscious casualty (b, fig 17), even though he may be conscious, to permit drainage from his mouth.

23. Sucking Wounds of the Chest

a. General. A chest wound which results in air being sucked into the chest cavity is particularly dangerous. The chest wound itself is not as dangerous as the air which goes through it into the chest cavity. This will cause the lung on the injured side to collapse (fig 59). The casualty's life may, therefore, depend upon how quickly you make the wound airtight.

b. Special Precautions, Procedures, and Modifications to A B C D Lifesaving Measures.

(1) Have the casualty forcibly exhale (breathe out), if possible, and hold his breath while you seal the wound.

(2) Seal the wound as follows:

(*a*) Apply the inside surface of the plastic wrapper which you take off the field first aid dressing directly over the wound; then press the first aid dressing firmly over this wrapper and have an assistant or the casualty exert pressure on the dressing with his open hand while you secure the bandages attached to the dressing around the casualty's body (fig 60). Be careful not to touch the inside of the plastic wrapper before placing it over the wound.

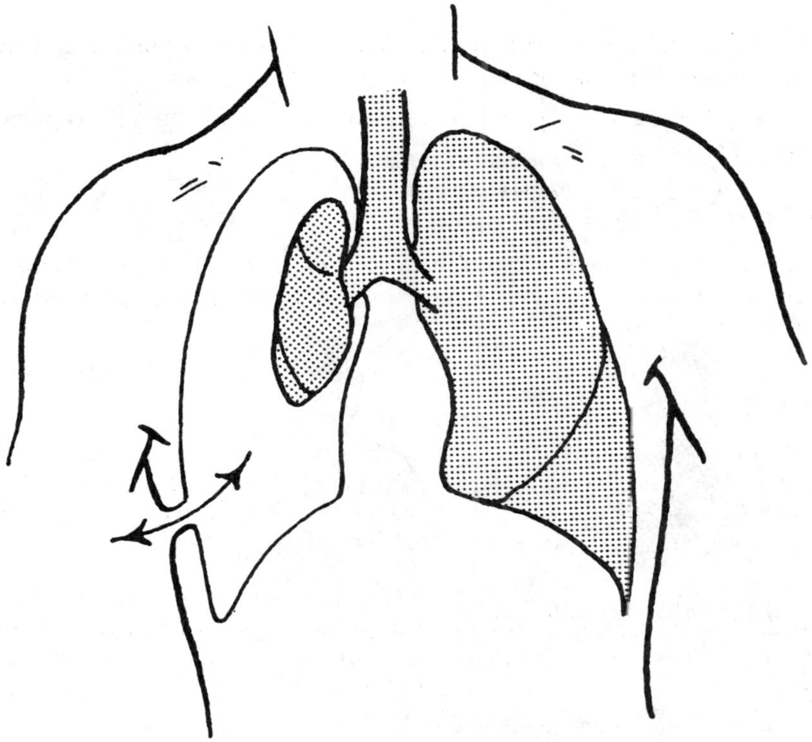

Figure 59. Sucking wound of the chest.

Note. If the field first aid dressing is packaged in a waterproof paper wrapper instead of a plastic wrapper, apply the inside surface of the metal foil side against the wound. If petroleum gauze is available (app B), it should be applied directly over the wound.

(*b*) Obtain a strip of bandaging material from clothing, a shelter half, a blanket, a poncho, et cetera, and apply it over the dressing and around the casualty's body to create further pressure, thus making the wound airtight. Each turn of this bandaging material must overlap the preceding one in order to provide firm, evenly distributed pressure over the entire dressing.

(*c*) Secure the bandages with a belt.

(3) If the casualty finds it more comfortable to sit up, allow him to do so. If he chooses to lie down, encourage him to lie on his injured side so that the lung on his uninjured side can receive more air. Also, the surface on which he is lying serves somewhat as a splint to the injured side and thus decreases pain.

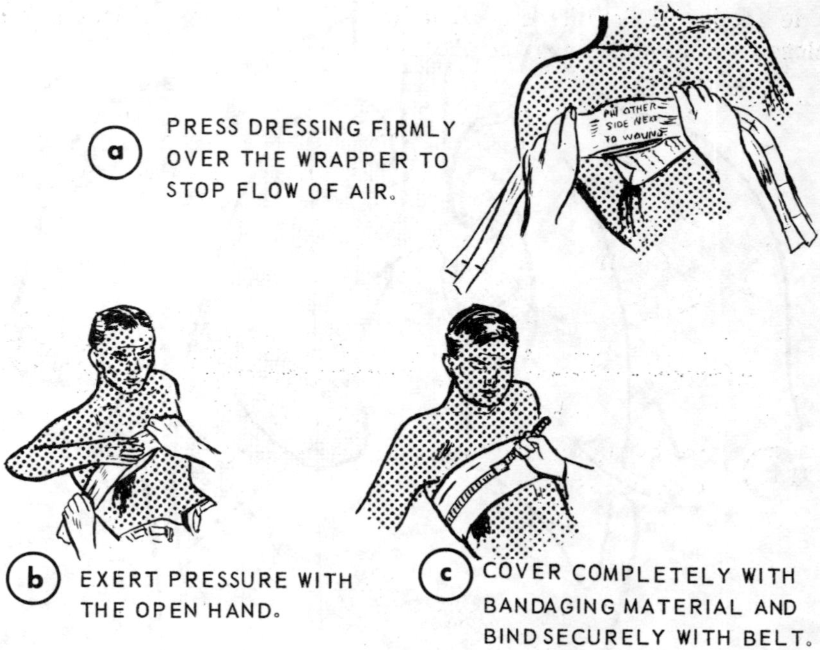

Figure 60. Sealing a sucking wound of the chest.

24. Abdominal Wounds

a. General. The most serious abdominal wound is one in which an object penetrates the abdominal wall and pierces internal organs or large blood vessels.

b. Special Precautions and Modifications to A B C D Lifesaving Measures (chap 2).

(1) Do not touch or try to push protruding organs such as intestines into the wound; apply one or more sterile dressings over them (a and b, fig 61). If it is necessary to move an exposed intestine onto the abdomen in order to cover the wound adequately; then do so. Secure the dressings in place with bandages (c, fig 61); but do not apply them tightly, as internal bleeding cannot be controlled by pressure and excessive pressure can cause additional injury.

(2) Do not give or allow the casualty to take anything by mouth, as it will eventually pass through the injured intestines and spread contamination in the abdomen. The casualty's lips may be moistened to help lessen his thirst.

(3) Leave the casualty on his back, but turn his head to one

side (c, fig 61). Since the casualty will likely vomit, watch him closely to prevent him from choking.

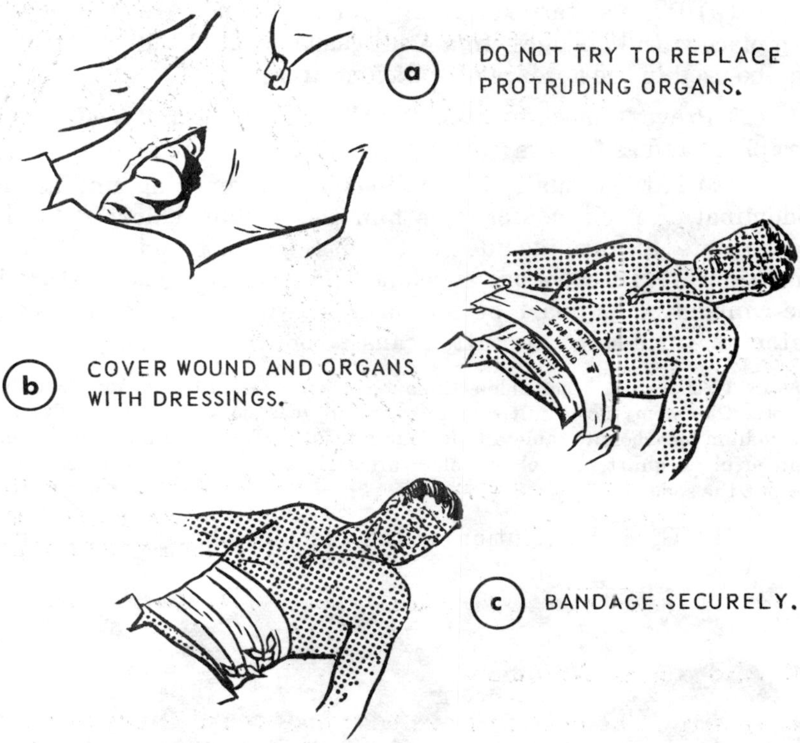

Figure 61. First aid for an abdominal wound.

25. Severe Burns

a. General. If a casualty has a burn which is blistered or charred, special first aid measures are required. The primary objective when giving first aid to a burned casualty is to prevent or lessen shock and infection.

b. Special Precautions, Procedures, and Modifications to A B C D Lifesaving Measures.

(1) Protect the burn against further contamination as follows, thus lessening the possibilities of infection.

(*a*) If clothing covers the burn, cut and lift it gently away without touching the burn.

1. Do not try to remove pieces of cloth which have stuck to the burn or to clean the burn in any way.

2. Do not pull clothes over the burned area.

3. Do not break blisters.

4. Do not put ointment or any medication whatsoever on the burn. For use of ointment on minor burns, see paragraph 34*b*.

(*b*) Place a sterile dressing over the burned area and secure it in place with bandages. In a mass casualty situation, clean sheet may be used in the absence of sufficient dressings.

(2) Prevent shock by applying the measures discussed in paragraph 14 and as follows:

(*a*) If the casualty is conscious, is not vomiting, and has no abdominal or neck wound, give him the sodium chloride-sodium bicarbonate mixture included in the first aid case and the Phase I Unit (app B). Dissolve one envelope (4.5 grams) of the mixture in one canteenful or quart of cool or cold water. Never use warm water, as warm salt water often causes vomiting.

Note. If the sodium chloride-sodium bicarbonate mixture is not available, dissolve four army issue salt tablets (one-half teaspoonful of loose salt) and two sodium bicarbonate tablets (one-fourth teaspoonful of baking soda) in one canteenful or quart of cool or cold water. If only salt is available, use it without the soda.

(*b*) Give the solution to the casualty slowly, having him

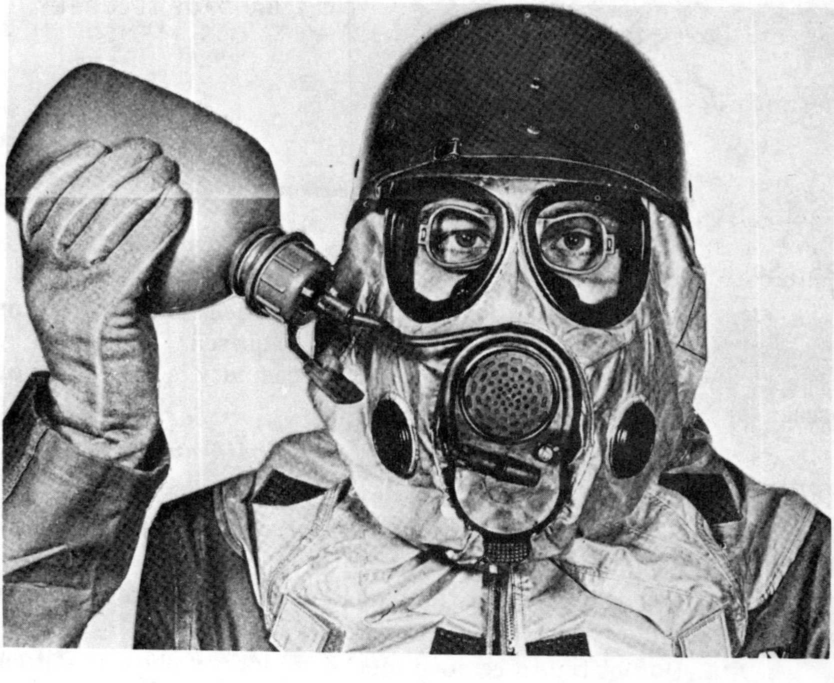

Figure 62. Administration of oral fluids in a toxic environment.

consume the entire amount over a 1-hour period. Should the casualty become nauseated, stop giving him the solution to prevent vomiting and further loss of fluids; but keep the solution available for him to drink later. This solution helps restore body fluids and salts which a burn casualty loses.

(*c*) If the casualty is wearing a protective mask (fig 62), turn the valve handle to the *right,* thus moving the drinking tube on the inside of his mask into his mouth; then insert the drinking tube on the outside of his mask into the MI Protective Canteen Cap on his canteen, making sure that a tight seal is effected. Tilt the canteen upward and then downward in the appropriate positions for the casualty to drink the solution described above.

Section II. FRACTURES

26. General

Fractures (broken bones) can cause total disability or death; on the other hand, they can more often be treated so that the casualty completely recovers from his injury. A great deal depends upon the first aid that the casualty receives before he is moved. First aid includes immobilization of the fractured part in addition to the application of lifesaving measures A B C D as required.

27. Kinds of Fractures

a. Closed Fracture. A closed fracture is a break in the bone without a break in the overlying skin; however there may be tissue damage beneath the skin. Even though an injury may be a dislocation or sprain, it should be considered as a closed fracture for purposes of applying first aid.

b. Open Fracture. An open fracture is a break in the bone as well as in the overlying skin. The broken bone may have come through the skin, or a missile such as a bullet or shell fragment may have gone through the flesh to the bone. An open fracture is subject to contamination.

28. Signs of a Fracture

A fracture is easily recognized when the bone is protruding through the skin, the part is in an unnatural position, or the chest wall is caved in. Other signs of a fracture are tenderness or pain when slight pressure is applied to the injured part and swelling as well as discoloration of the skin at the site of the injury. Deep, sharp pain upon an attempt to move the part is also a sign of a

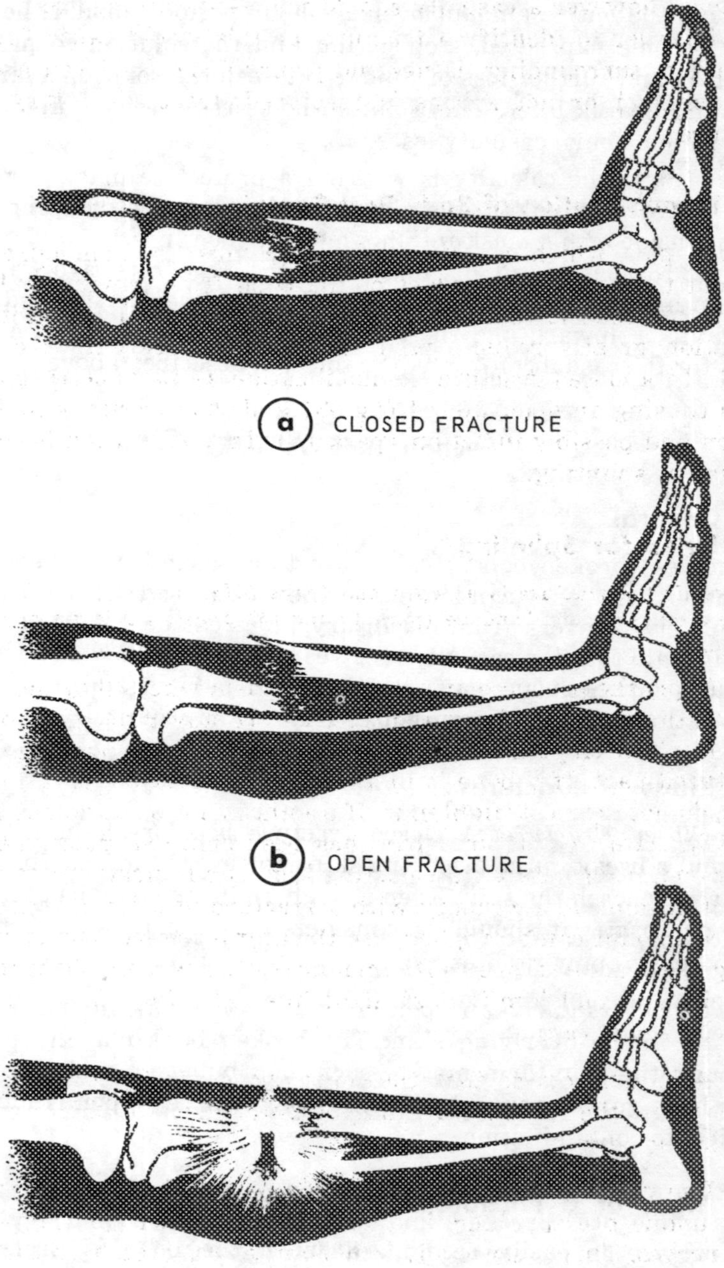

Figure 63. Kinds of fractures.

fracture; however a casualty should not be encouraged to move a part in order to identify a fracture, as this would cause further damage to surrounding tissues and promote shock. If you are not sure whether or not a bone is fractured, treat the injury as a fracture.

29. Immobilization of Body Part Containing a Fracture

A body part which contains a fracture must be immobilized to prevent the razor-sharp edges of the bone from moving and cutting tissue, muscle, blood vessels, and nerves. Furthermore, immobilization greatly reduces pain and helps to prevent or control shock. In a closed fracture, immobilization keeps bone fragments from causing an open wound (fig 63) and thus prevents contamination and possibly infection (para 15). Immobilization is accomplished by splinting.

30. Rules for Splinting

Note. If the fracture is an open one (para 27*b*), first stop the bleeding, apply a dressing, and bandage (para 10 and 15) as you would for any other wound.

a. Apply the proven principle "Splint them where they lie." This means to splint the fractured part before any movement of the casualty is attempted and without any change in the position of the fractured part. If a bone is in an unnatural position or a joint is bent, do not try to straighten it. If a joint is not bent, do not try to bend it. After a fractured part has been splinted, place the casualty on a litter before transporting him. If circumstances make it essential to move a casualty with a fracture of a lower extremity before a splint can be applied, use the uninjured leg as a splint by tying the fractured one to it; then grasp the casualty beneath the armpits and pull him in a straight line only. Do not roll him or move him sideways.

b. Apply splints so that the joint above the fracture and the joint below the fracture are immobilized. Place a splint on each side of the part.

c. Use padding between the injured part and the splint to prevent undue pressure and further injury to tissue, blood vessels, and nerves. This is especially important at the crotch, in the armpit, and on places where the splints come in contact with bony parts such as the elbow, wrist, knee, and ankle joint.

d. Bind splints securely with bandages at several points above and below the fracture but do not bind tightly enough to interfere with the flow of blood. Tie bandages with a square knot and let the knot be on the outer splint.

e. Support a splintered arm which is bent at the elbow with a sling. A sling is also used to support a sprained arm or an arm with a painful wound.

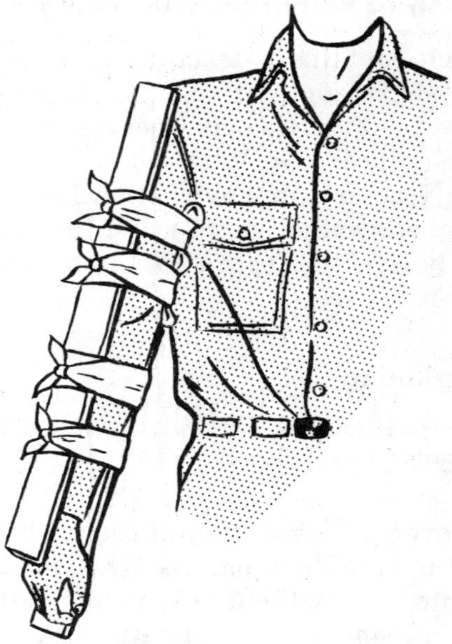

Figure 64. Board splints applied to fractured arm or elbow when elbow is not bent.

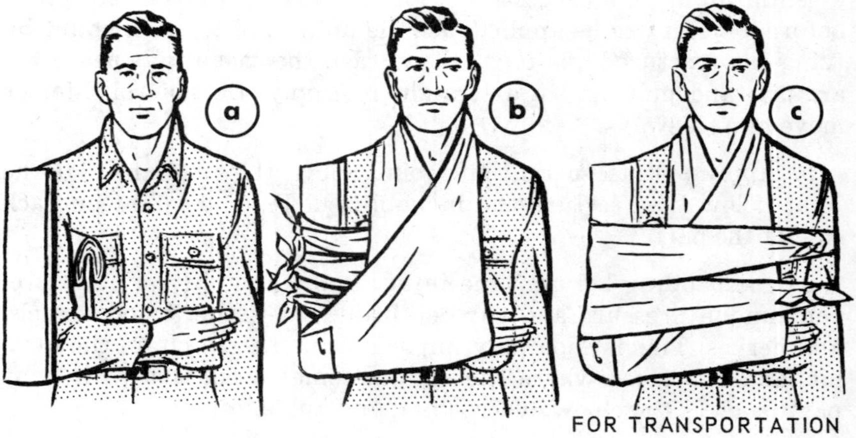

Figure 65. Fractured upper arm splinted with boards and supported with sling and cravat.

31. Splints, Padding, Bandages, and Slings

a. Splints. Splints may be improvised from such items as boards, poles, sticks, tree limbs, carbines, rifles, rolled magazines or newspapers, and cardboard. The wire ladder splint is provided in the fracture pack of the Phase I Unit (app B). This splint may be bent as required to fit the part. Also, two of these splints may be overlapped and fastened together to obtain the desired length. Roller bandage (fig 22) may be applied in a specific way to immobilize certain body parts such as the collarbone and shoulder. If nothing is available for a splint, the chest wall can be used to immobilize a

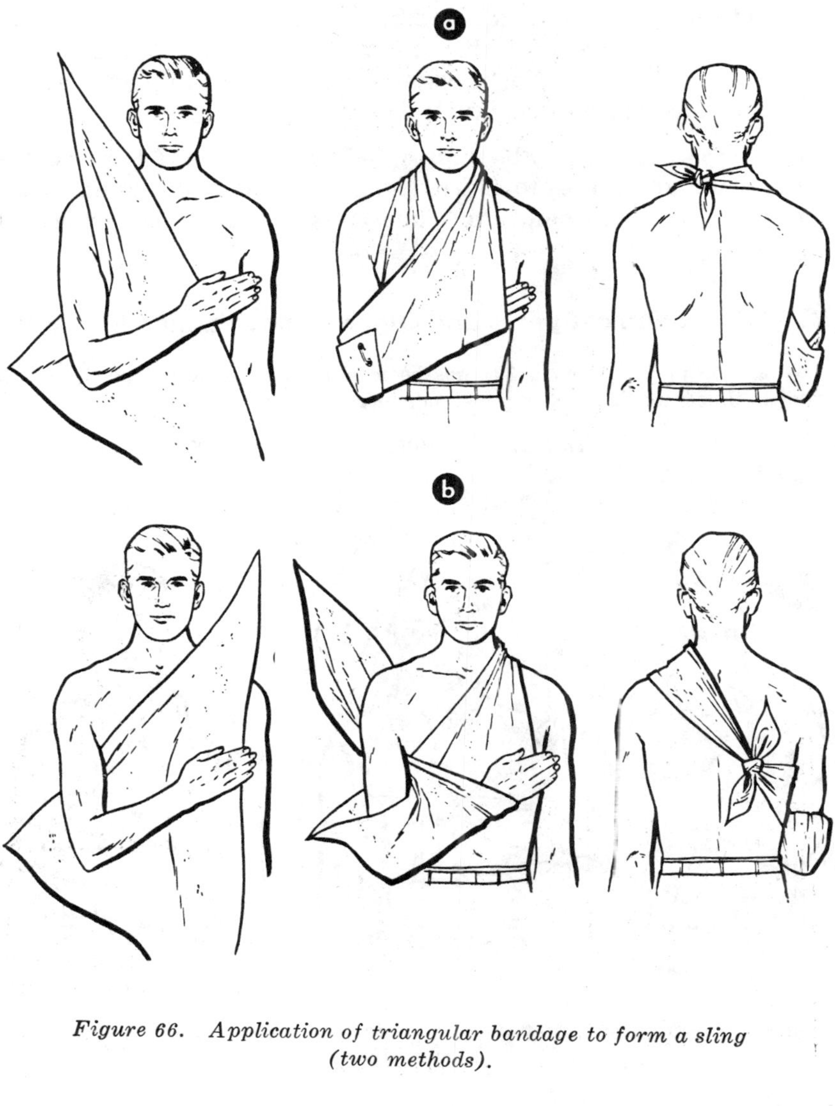

Figure 66. Application of triangular bandage to form a sling (two methods).

fractured arm; and the uninjured leg can be used to immobilize, to some extent, a fractured leg.

***Caution:* If weapons are used as splints, be absolutely sure they are unloaded.**

b. Padding. Padding may be improvised from a jacket, blanket, poncho, shelter half or leafy vegetation. Cotton wadding is provided in the fracture pack of the Phase I Unit (app B).

c. Bandages. Bandages may be improvised from belts, rifle slings, bandoleers, and handkerchiefs and from strips torn from such items as clothing and blankets. The triangular bandage (fig 21) and the roller bandage (fig 22) are provided in some first aid kits and in the Phase I Unit (app B). Narrow materials such as wire or cord should not be used to secure a splint in place. No ties should be made across the break.

d. Slings. Slings may be improvised by using the tail of a coat or shirt, belts, and pieces torn from such items as clothing and blankets. The triangular bandage (*c* above) is ideal for this purpose.

32. Application of Splints and Other Immobilization Methods

Note. The padding (para 30) has been omitted in some of the figures in order to illustrate the splinting methods more clearly.

a. Splints and Slings for Fractures of the Upper Extremities (fig 64–69).

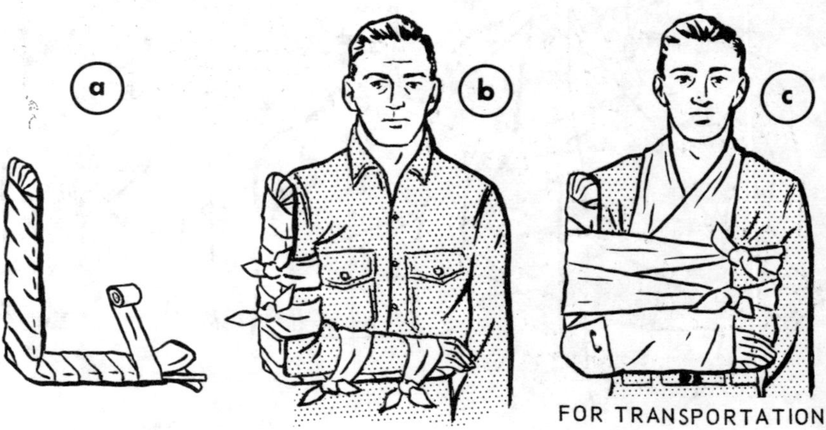

Figure 67. Wire ladder splint applied to fractured arm or elbow when elbow is bent.

b. Splints for Fractures of the Lower Extremities (fig 70–73)

c. Immobilization of Fractured Jaw, Collarbone, Shoulder, and Ribs.

(1) Apply a cravat (para 18*b*) or roller bandage (para 18*c*) to immobilize a fractured jaw as illustrated in figures 35 and 36.

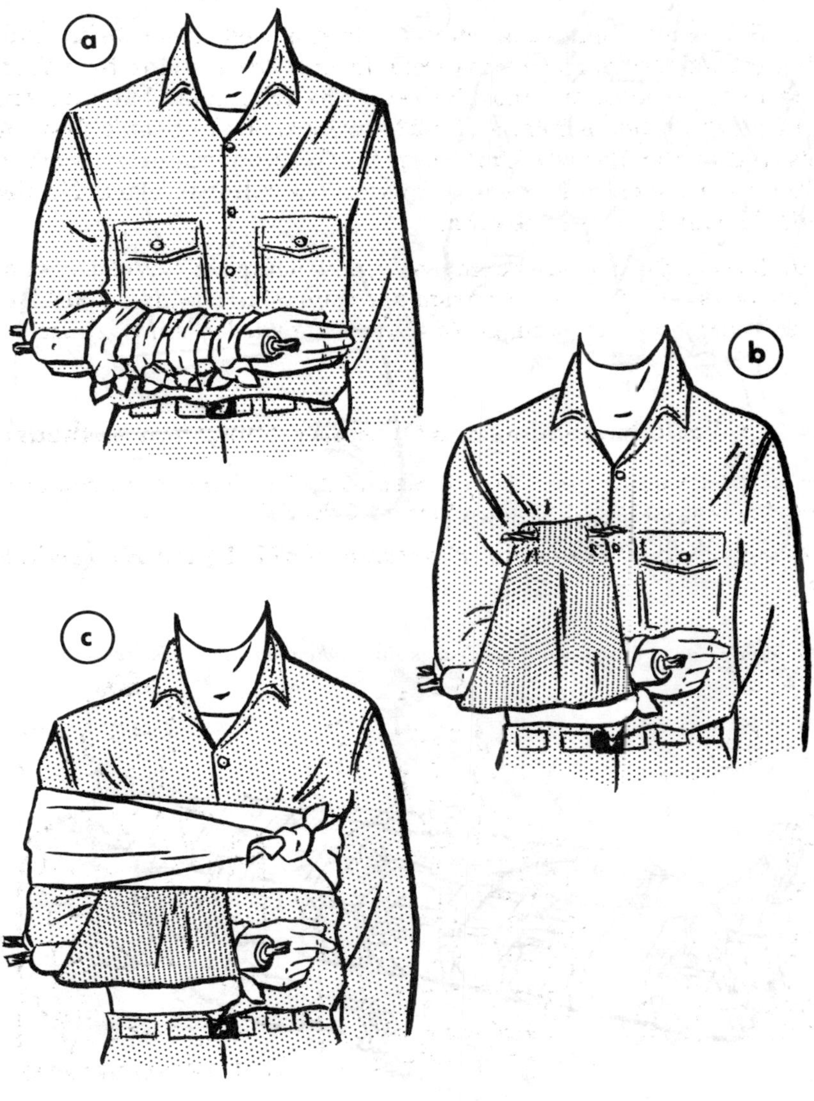

Figure 68. Fractured forearm or wrist splintered with sticks and supported with tail of shirt and strip of material.

Direct all bandaging support to the top of the casualty's head and not to the back of his neck, as the latter pulls the jaw back, thus interfering with his breathing.

(2) Apply two belts, two cravats (para 18*b*), or roller bandage (para 18*c*) to immobilize a fractured collarbone, using the figure-of-eight technique as illustrated in figures 74 and 75.

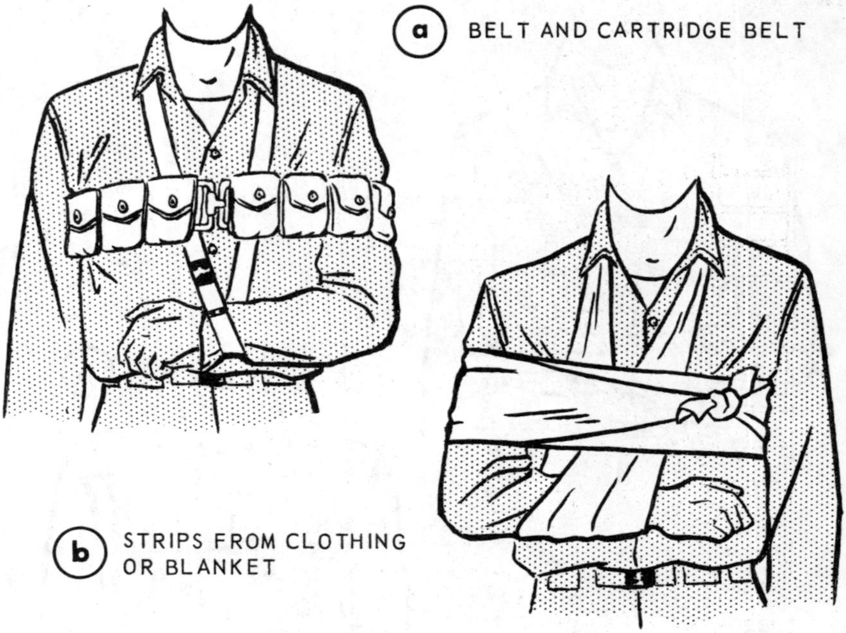

Figure 69. Chest wall used as splint when no splint is available.

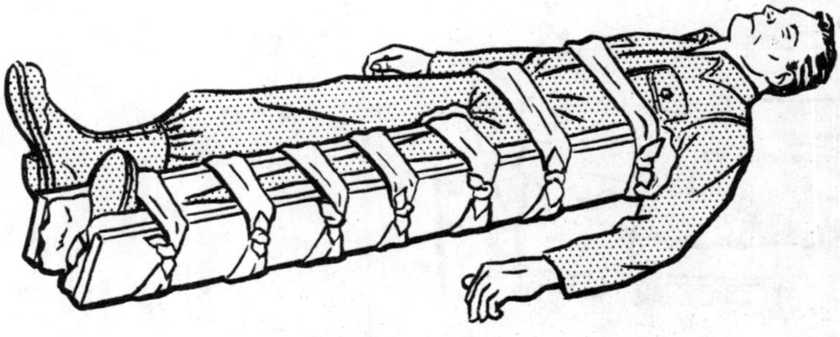

Figure 70. Board splints applied to lower extremity.

(3) Apply two cravats (para 18*b*) or roller bandage (para 18*c*) to immobilize a fractured or dislocated shoulder, using the techniques illustrated in figures 76 and 77.

(4) Apply three cravats (para 18*b*) to immobilize fractured ribs as illustrated in figure 78. The cravats should be applied upon exhalation of air from the lungs and tied on the side opposite the fracture.

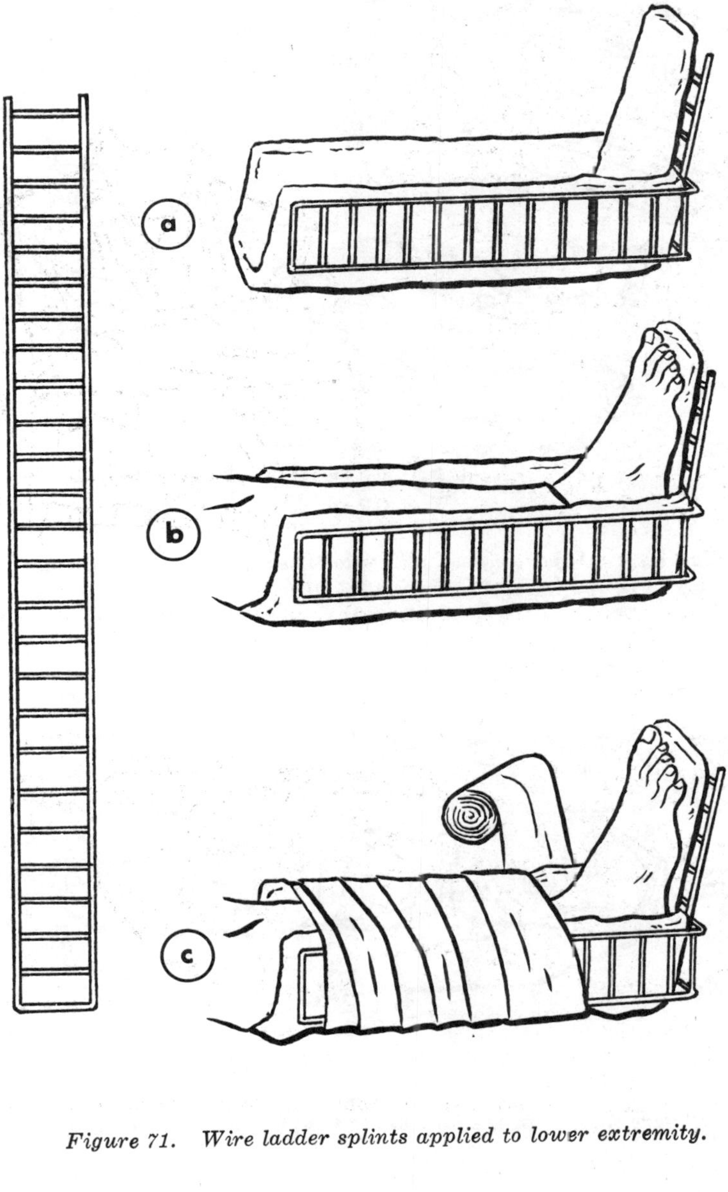

Figure 71. Wire ladder splints applied to lower extremity.

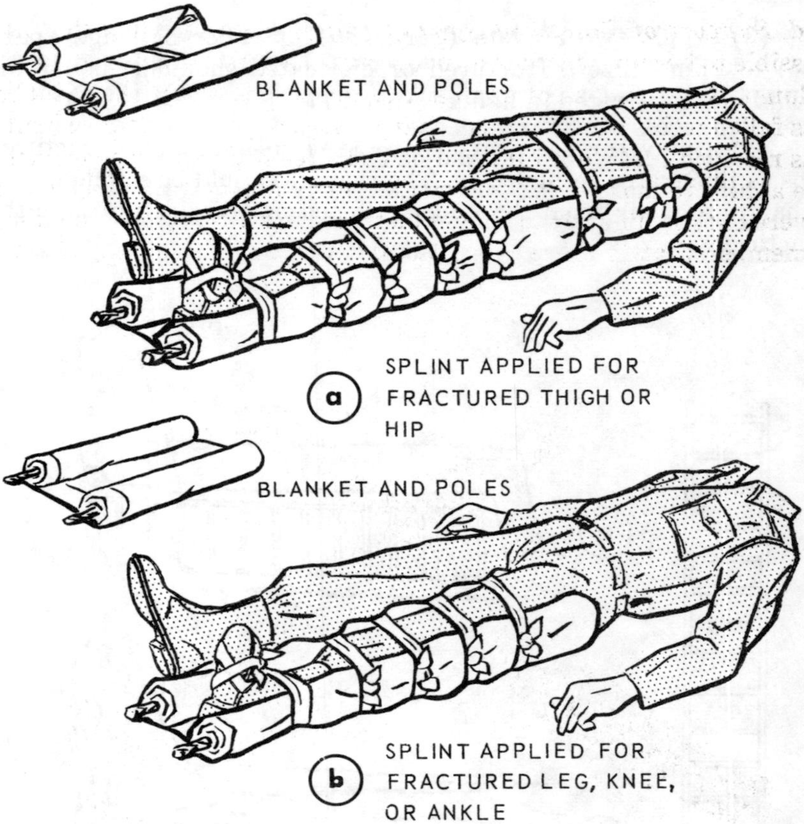

Figure 72. Application of splints to lower extremity, using poles rolled in a blanket.

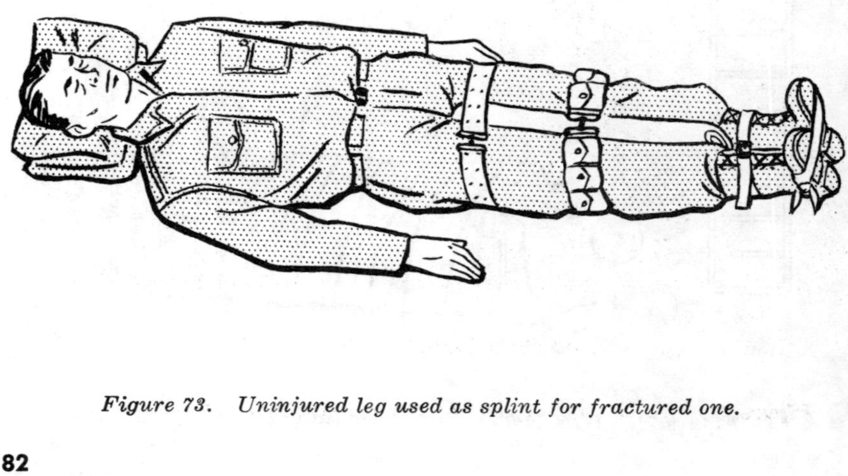

Figure 73. Uninjured leg used as splint for fractured one.

d. Support of Fractured Spinal Column (Back). It is often impossible to be sure whether or not a casualty has a fractured spinal column. Be suspicious of any back injury, especially if the casualty has fallen or his back has been sharply struck or bent. If a casualty has received such an injury and he lacks feeling in his legs or lacks the ability to move them, you can be reasonably sure that he has a severe back injury which should be treated as a fracture. You must remember that if there is a fracture, bending the spinal column

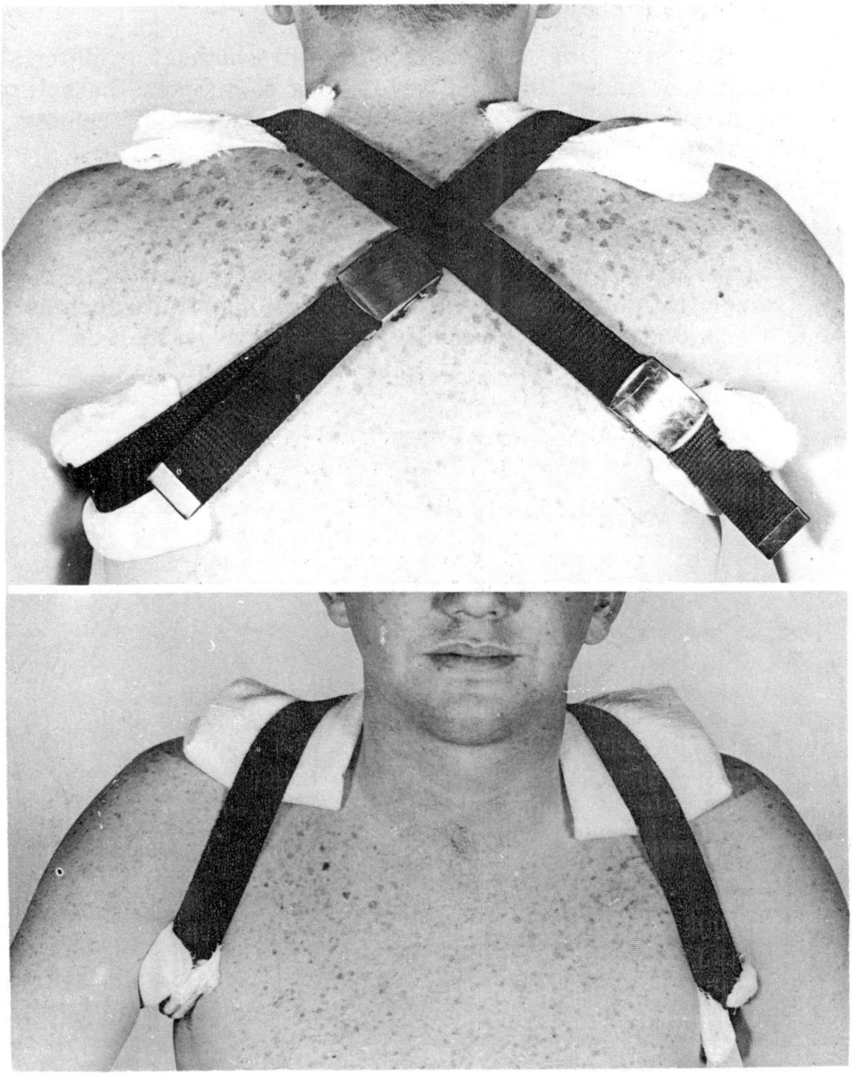

Figure 74. ***Application of belts to immobilize a fractured collarbone.***

can cause the sharp bone fragments to bruise or cut the spinal cord, resulting in permanent paralysis. The spinal column must maintain a sway-back position to remove pressure from the spinal cord (fig 79).

(1) *Steps to follow if the casualty is not to be transported until medical personnel arrive.*

(*a*) If the casualty is conscious, caution him not to move.

(*b*) Leave the casualty in the position in which he is found. Do not move any body part.

(*c*) If he is lying with his face up, slip a blanket or material of similar size under the arch of his back to support the spinal column in a sway-back position. If he is lying with his face down, do not put anything under any part of his body.

(2) *Steps to follow if the casualty must be transported before medical personnel arrive.*

(*a*) *Face-up position.* If the casualty is lying with his face up, transportation must be by litter or a firm substitute such as a wide board longer than the casualty is tall. Tie the casualty's hand over his waistline with a cravat or strip of cloth and lay a folded

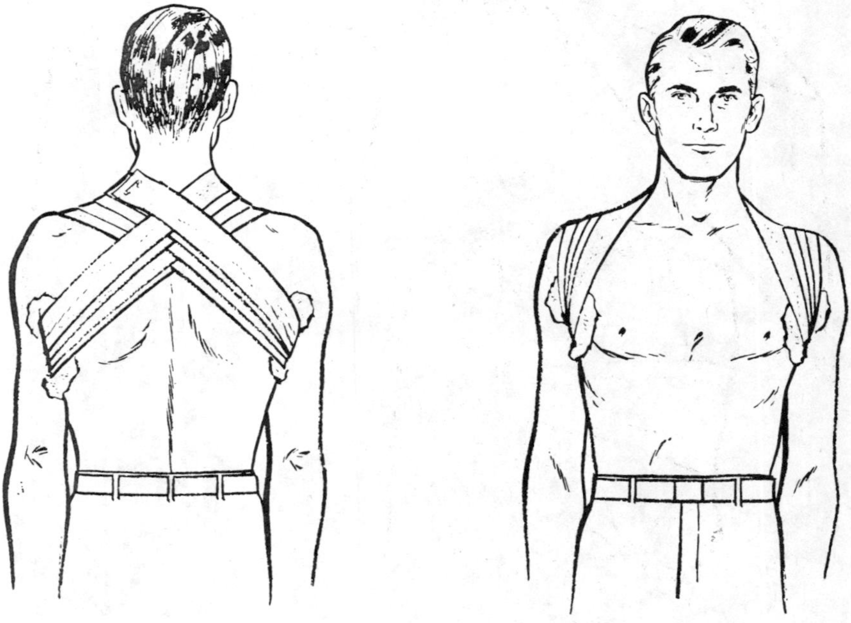

Figure 75. Application of roller bandage to immobilize a fractured collarbone (figure-of-eight technique).

blanket across the litter where the arch of the casualty's back is to be placed. Using a four-man team (fig 80), place the casualty on the litter without bending his spinal column:

1. Kneeling on the knee nearer the casualty's feet, No. 2, 3, and 4 men position themselves on one side of the casualty. No. 1 man positions himself on the opposite side. No. 2, 3, and 4 place

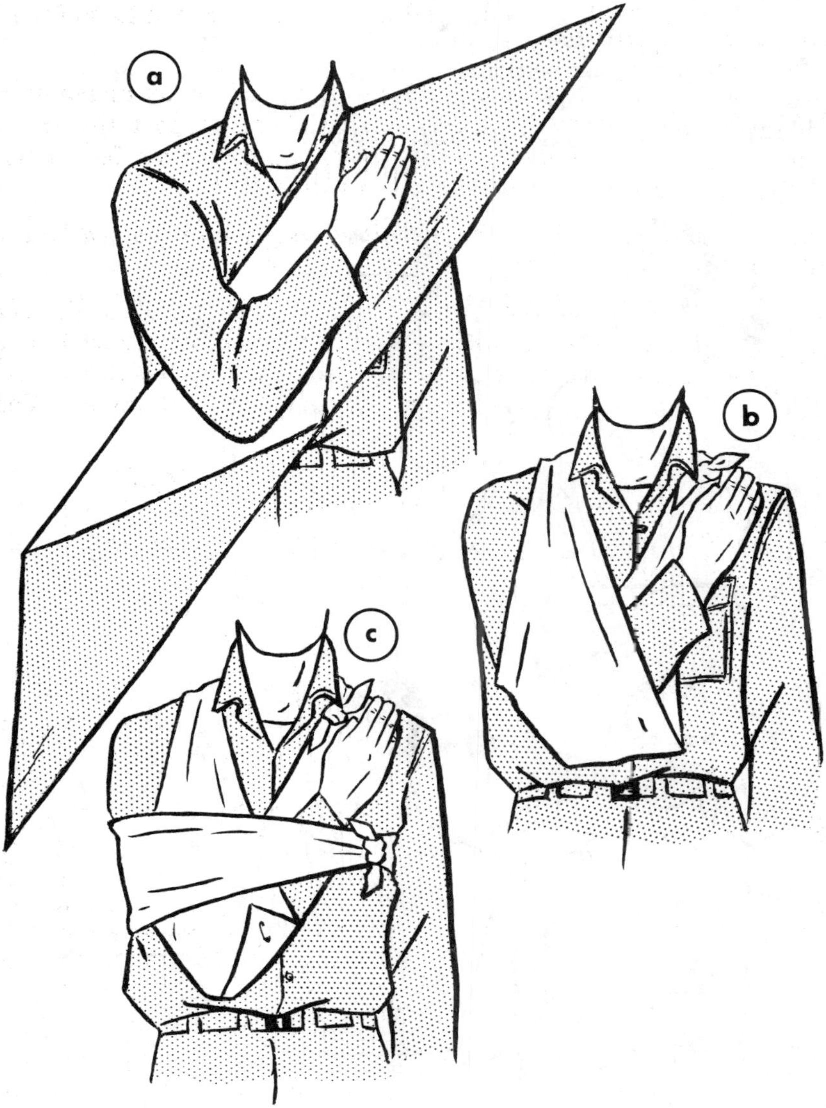

Figure 76. Application of cravats to immobilize a fractured or dislocated shoulder.

their hand as illustrated in figure 80. No. 1 assists in lifting at the site of the fracture.

2. All men in close coordination gently lift the casualty about 8 inches; then No. 1 slides the litter under the casualty, insures that the blanket is in proper position, and returns to his original position.

3. All men in close coordination gently lower the casualty onto the litter.

(*b*) *Face-down position.* If the casualty is lying with his face down, he must be transported in this same position. Using the four-man team ((*a*) above), lift him onto a regular litter or a blanket roll litter (para 47*c*), keeping the spinal column in a

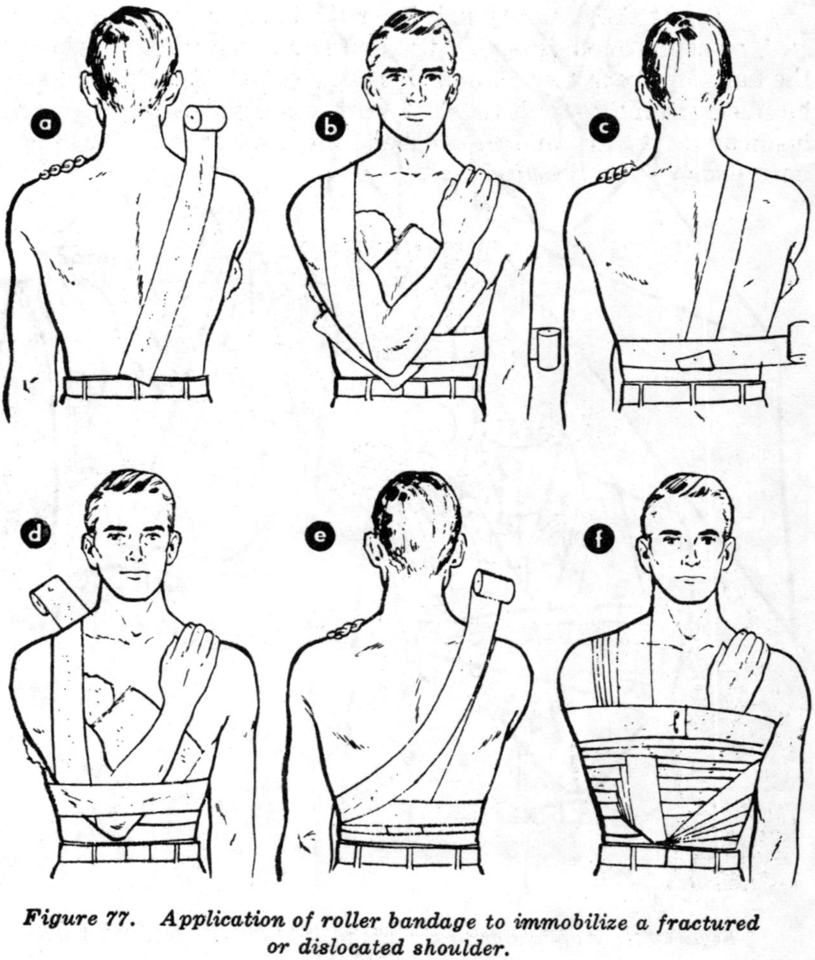

***Figure 77.** Application of roller bandage to immobilize a fractured or dislocated shoulder.*

sway-back position. If a regular litter is to be used, first place a folded blanket on the litter at the point where the chest will be placed.

e. Immobilization of Fractured Neck. A fractured neck is extremely dangerous. Bone fragments may bruise or cut the spinal cord just as in the case of a fractured back.

(1) *Steps to follow if the casualty is not to be transported until medical personnel arrive.*

(*a*) If the casualty is conscious, caution him not to move. Moving may cause death.

(*b*) Leave the casualty in the position in which he is found. If the neck is in an abnormal position, immobilize it in this position ((*d*) below).

(*c*) If the casualty is lying with his face up, keep his head still, raise his shoulders slightly, and slip a roll of cloth which has the bulk of a bath towel under his neck (a, fig 81). The roll should be thick enough to arch the neck only slightly, leaving the back of his head on the ground. Do not bend the neck or head forward. Do not raise or twist the head.

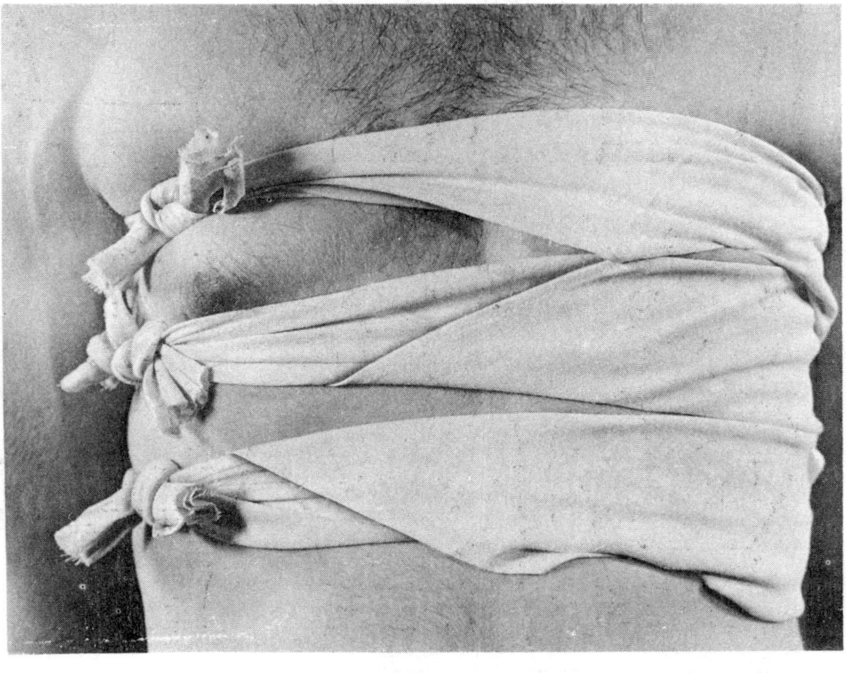

Figure 78. Application of cravats to immobilize fractured ribs on the left side.

(*d*) Immobilize the casualty's head (b, fig 81). This may be accomplished by padding heavy objects such as rocks or the casualty's boots and placing them on each side of his head. If it is necessary to use the casualty's boots, they should first be filled with stones, gravel, sand, or dirt and tied tightly at the top. It may be necessary to stuff pieces of material in the tops of the boots to secure the contents.

(2) *Steps to follow if the casualty must be prepared for transportation before medical personnel arrive.* The services of at least two persons are necessary to prepare a casualty with a fractured neck for transportation because the head and trunk must be moved in unison. The two persons must work in close coordination to avoid bending the neck in any way. The proper procedure is described as follows:

(*a*) Place a wide board lengthwise beside the casualty. It should extend at least 4 inches beyond his head and feet (a, fig 82).

(*b*) If the casualty is lying with his face up, No. 1 man steadies the casualty's head and neck between his hands while No. 2 man with one foot and one knee placed against the board to prevent it from slipping grasps the casualty at his shoulder and hip and gently slides him onto the board (b, fig 82).

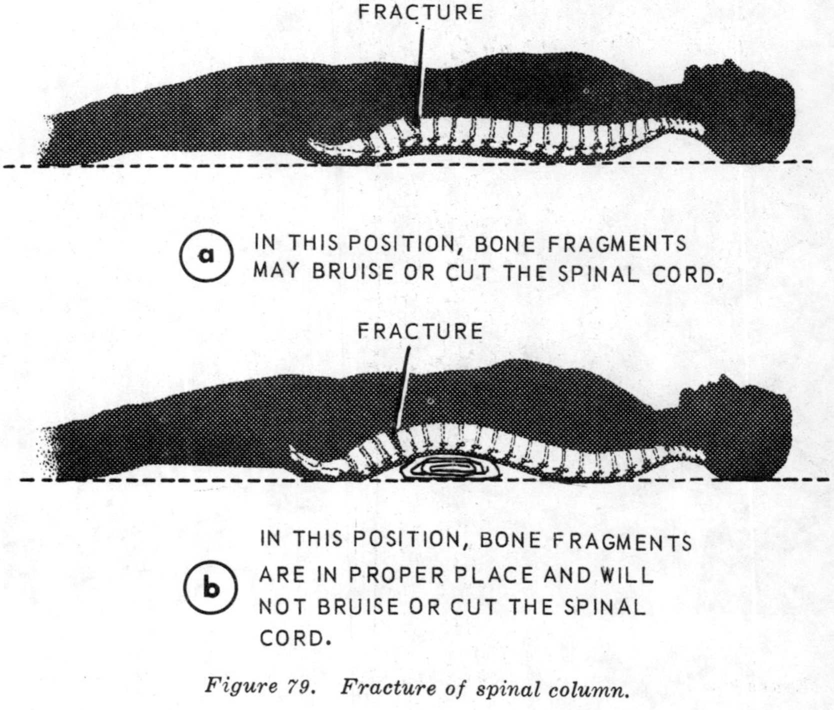

Figure 79. Fracture of spinal column.

(*c*) If the casualty is lying with his face down, No. 1 man steadies the casualty's head and neck between his hands while No. 2 man gently rolls him over onto the board (c, fig 82).

(*d*) No. 1 man continues to steady the casualty's head and neck while No. 2 man raises his shoulders slightly, places padding under his neck ((1) (*c*) above), and immobilizes his head. The head may be immobilized with his boots (b, fig 81), with stones rolled in pieces of blanket or other material (d, fig 82), or with wire ladder splints (f, fig 82) as available (app B). If wire ladder splints are used, two of them are overlapped, fastened together, shaped to fit

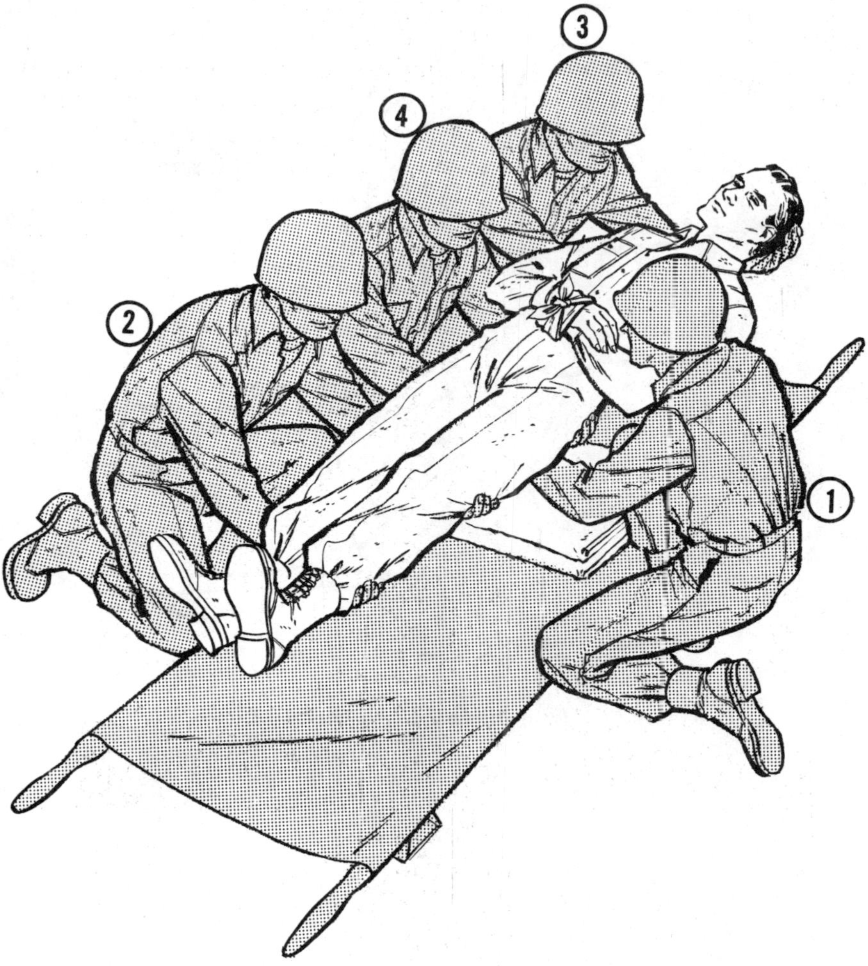

Figure 80. Placing a casualty with fractured spinal column onto a litter.

the head and shoulders, padded, positioned, and secured with bandages which are extended under the armpits and over the shoulders, under the head and across the chin, and under the head and across the forehead (f, fig 82).

(*e*) Secure any improvised supports ((*d*) above) in position with a cravat or strip of cloth extended across the casualty's forehead and under the board (e, fig 82).

(*f*) Lift the board onto a litter or blanket, as available, to transport him.

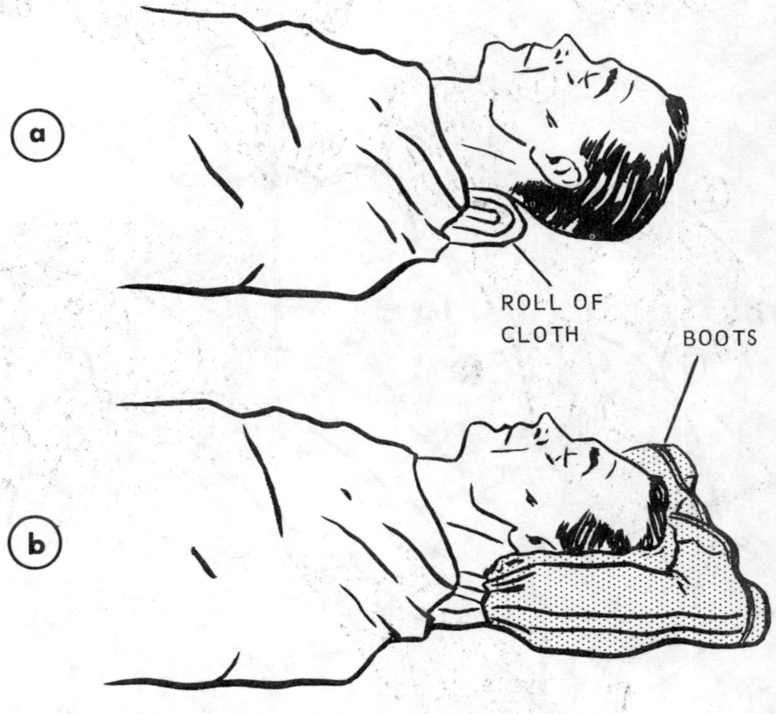

Figure 81. Immobilization of a fractured neck.

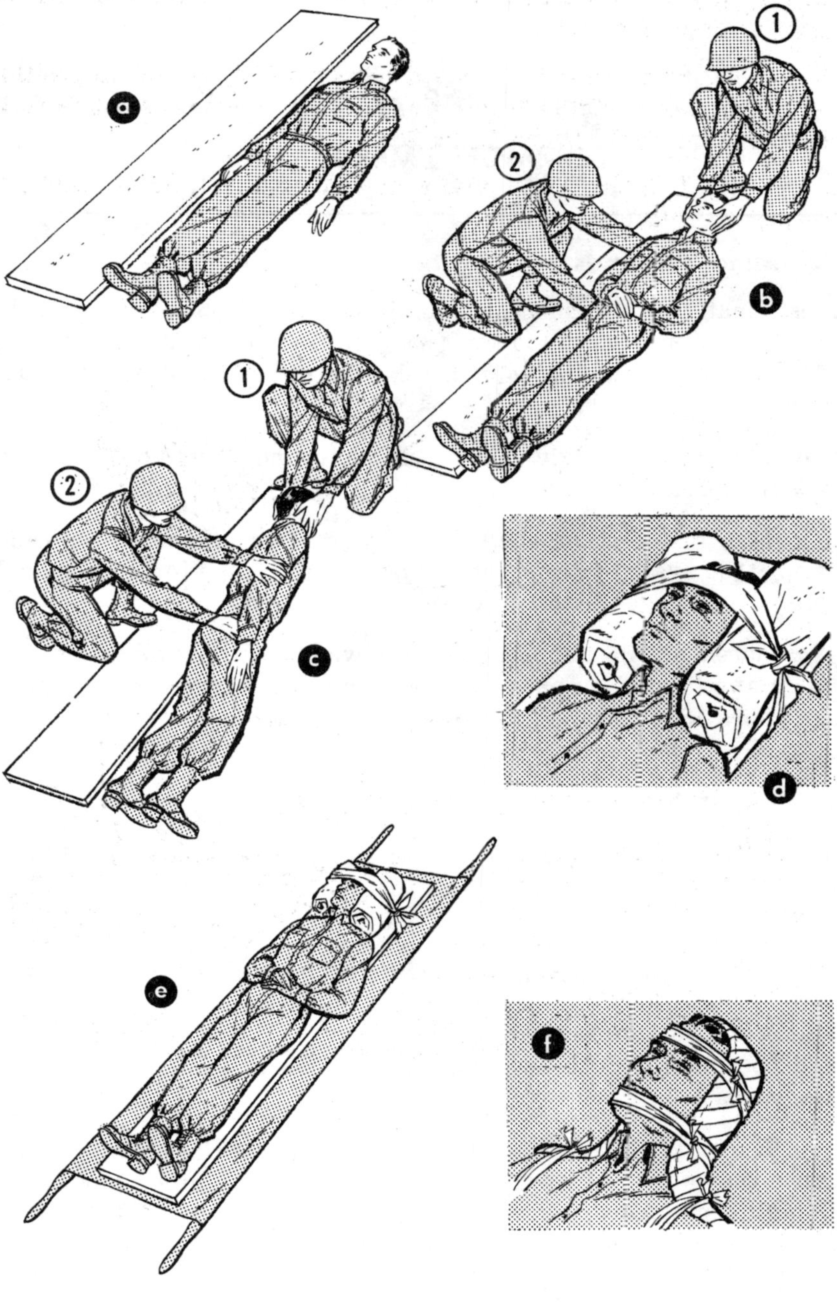

Figure 82. Preparation of a casualty with a fractured neck for transportation.

CHAPTER 4

COMMON EMERGENCIES

33. Minor Wounds

Most small wounds, such as cuts, do not usually bleed very much. Infection from contamination (para 15*a*) is the principal danger. If you receive a minor wound, take the following first aid measures:

a. Do not allow anything to touch the wound, except as described in *b* and *c* below.

b. If a disinfectant such as Tincture Benzalkonium Chloride (app B) is available, apply it to the wound. (In no instance should solutions stronger than 1:1000 or 1:750 be used.)

c. Place a sterile compress over the wound without allowing it to touch anything else (para 16) and secure it in place with a bandage (para 18).

34. Minor Burns

Minor burns may be caused by exposure to dry heat, hot liquids, chemicals, electricity, or rays of the sun. Minor burns are of two types:

a. *Small Burns Which Include Blistering or Charring*. Since the skin is most likely to break when it is blistered or charred, cover it with a sterile compress (para 17) to protect it from contamination and possible infection. Secure the compress in place with a bandage (para 18).

b. *Burns With No Blistering or Charring*. If the burn does not cause the skin to blister, char, or break, it is a minor burn even though it may cover a large area of the body, as in mild sunburn. It is not necessary to cover such a burn with sterile compress. The lubricant in Phase I Unit (app B) may be applied in a thin layer to relieve pain. Do not apply this lubricant to a burn in which the skin is blistered, charred, or broken.

35. Foreign Body in the Eye

a. If a foreign particle gets into the eye, do not rub the eye. If the particle is beneath the upper eyelid, grasp the eyelashes of the upper lid and pull the lid up and away from contact with the surface of the eyeball. Hold the eyelid in this manner until tears flow freely. The tears will frequently flush out the particle. If this technique fails, attempt to remove it as shown in figure 83.

b. If the foreign particle is glass or metal or it cannot be removed by the techniques described in *a* above and illustrated in figure 83, bandage both of the casualty's eyes (para 19*b*) and get him to a medical treatment facility.

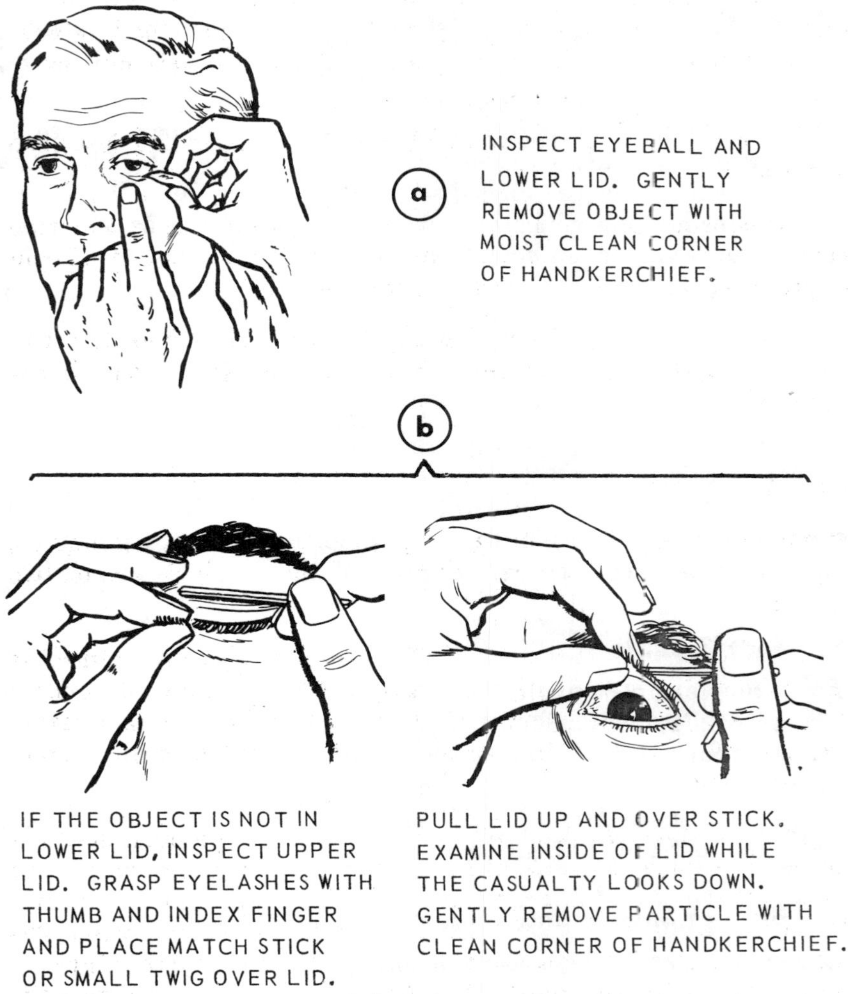

Figure 83. Removing a foreign particle from the eye.

Note. For very minimal injuries, bandaging only one eye may suffice. For any major injury, or in case of any doubt, both eyes must be bandaged. If only one eye is bandaged, the casualty will use his unaffected eye. Since eye movements are synchronized, use of the unaffected eye may result in movement of the affected one, thereby subjecting it to further injury.

c. If caustic or irritating material, such as battery acid, or ammonia, gets into the eye, immediately flush it with a large volume of water. To flush the right eye, turn the head to the right side; to flush the left eye, turn the head to the left side. This prevents the caustic or irritating material from being washed into the other eye.

36. Foreign Body in the Ear, Nose, or Throat

a. Never probe in an attempt to remove a foreign body from the ear. An insect in the ear may be removed simply by attracting it with a flashlight held to the ear. If this fails, it may be drowned or immobilized by pouring water into the ear. Foreign objects in the ear can sometimes be flushed out with water. However, if the object is something which will swell when wet, such as a seed or particle of wood, do not pour water into the ear.

b. Probing into the nose will generally jam a foreign object tighter. Damage to the nasal passages can also result. Try to remove the object by gently blowing the nose. If this fails, seek medical aid.

c. Coughing will frequently dislodge a foreign object from the throat. If this fails and the object can be reached, try to remove it with the fingers; but be careful to avoid pushing it farther down the throat. There is great danger of respiratory obstruction if the object cannot be removed, so get medical aid as quickly as possible.

37. Foot Trouble

Foot trouble can be avoided by taking proper care of the feet as discussed FM 21–10. Should you develop foot trouble such as a callus or corn, a blister, or athlete's foot, get medical aid. Do not cut a callus or corn, as this can cause a serious infection. If a blister develops and medical aid is not available, follow the first aid measure illustrated in figure 84.

38. Bites of Snakes and Spiders and Stings of Scorpions

Bites from snakes, black widow spiders, and brown recluse spiders and stings from scorpions can be prevented by following the measures discussed in FM 21–10. Should a person receive a bite or sting

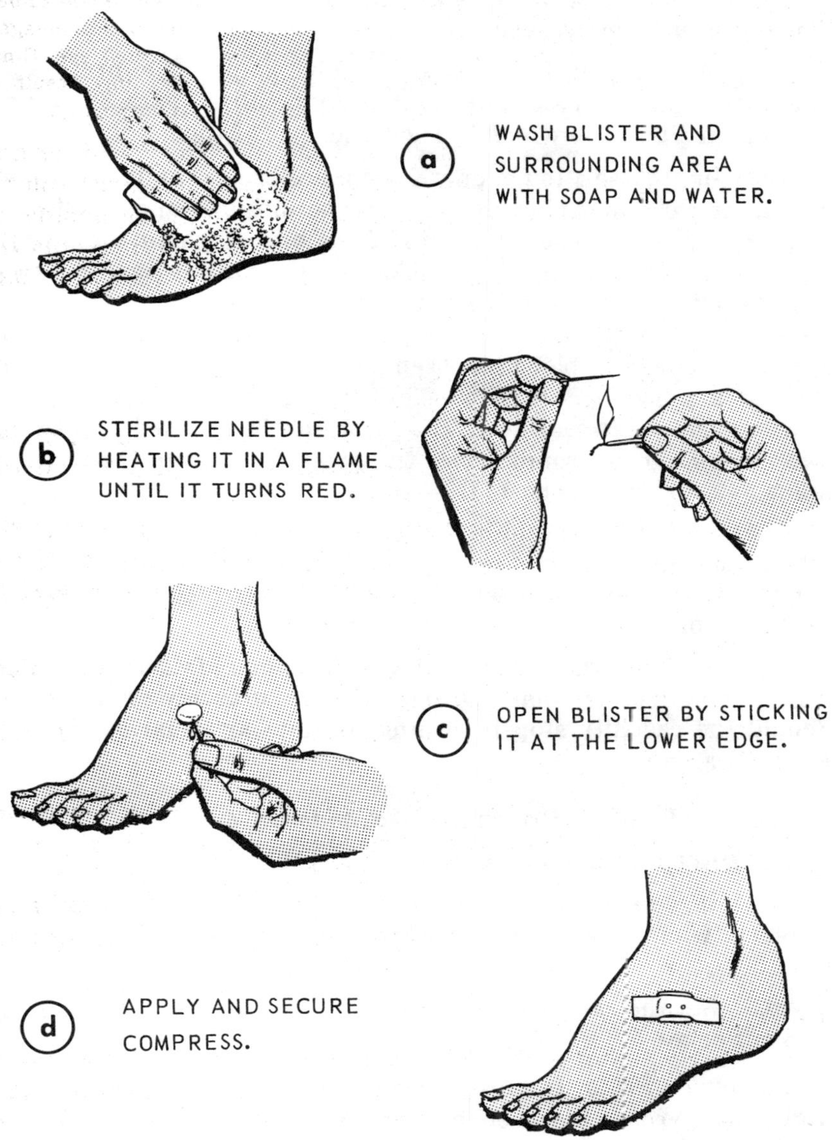

Figure 84. First aid for a blister.

from one of these venomous animals, the first aid measures outlined below should be followed.

a. Snake Bite.

(1) Keep the casualty as quiet as possible. Do not allow him to walk or run. If you can, kill and keep the snake so that it can be

identified to aid medical personnel in determining the proper antivenom serum for the casualty.

(2) Make the casualty as comfortable as possible, preferably in a sitting position, and immediately immobilize (para 32) a bitten limb in a position which is below the level of the heart.

(3) Improvise a tourniquet from a necktie, a handkerchief, or a strip of cloth and place it between the bite site and heart at a point 2 to 4 inches above the site of the bite. Tighten the tourniquet enough to stop the flow of blood in the vessels near the skin surface but not tight enough to stop the arterial flow or the pulse. As soon as the veins under the skin stand out prominently, the appropriate flow of blood has been properly halted. Also, the presence of a pulse in the part below the tourniquet indicates the continuance of arterial flow. The pulse can be checked by placing two fingers, not the thumb, over the pressure point in the wrist or ankle as appropriate (fig 14).

(4) Since medical aid is urgent in all cases of poisonous snake bite, send someone to summon assistance. If a litter or a vehicle is available, transport the casualty to the nearest medical treatment facility at once.

(5) Observe the casualty closely for signs of difficult breathing, as some types of snake poison affect the breathing mechanism. Should the casualty stop breathing, initiate artificial respiration (para 8) at once.

b. Black Widow or Brown Recluse Spider Bite.

(1) Keep the casualty as quiet as possible.

(2) If ice is available, place an ice pack around the region of the body where the bite occurred to keep the venom from spreading.

(3) Get the casualty to the nearest medical treatment facility without delay.

c. Scorpion Sting. In most areas of the world, scorpions are not highly dangerous; however in South America, Mexico, the Middle East, and some parts of North Africa, certain types can cause death if proper treatment is not administered.

(1) For an ordinary scorpion sting, put a piece of ice, if available, on the site of the sting as soon as possible. This may decrease the absorption of the venom by the body. Baking soda applied as a paste to the site of the bite will often relieve the pain.

(2) If the site of the sting is on the face, neck, or genital organs or if the sting is from a scorpion in the areas of the world

mentioned above, keep the casualty as quiet as possible and get him to the nearest medical treatment facility without delay.

39. Skin Eruptions from Poisonous Plants

In some persons the sap or juice of certain plants will cause skin eruptions. The most common plants are poison ivy, poison oak, and poison sumac. Skin eruptions from these plants can be prevented by learning how to identify the plants and by taking the proper control measures (FM 21–10). Should you develop a skin eruption several days after possible exposure to any of these plants, avoid scratching it and seek medical aid. The skin eruption first appears as redness and swelling accompanied by severe burning and itching; blisters appear later.

40. Conditions Caused by Extreme Heat

Conditions caused by extreme heat are heat exhaustion, heatstroke, and heat cramps, as well as sunburn and prickly heat. These conditions can be prevented by proper acclimatization to heat, adequate consumption of water and salt, and consistent practice of the prescribed preventive measures (FM 21–10).

a. Heat Exhaustion. This condition is caused by excessive loss of water and salt from the body. The symptoms of heat exhaustion are headache, excessive sweating, weakness, dizziness, and muscle cramps. Also, the skin is pale, cool, moist, and clammy. Heat exhaustion may come on gradually or suddenly. A victim of heat exhaustion should be given first aid as follows:

(1) Lay the casualty in a cool shaded area and loosen his clothing.

(2) If the casualty is conscious, give him cool salt water to drink. Prepare the salt water by dissolving two crushed salt tablets (one-fourth teaspoonful of table salt) in a canteen (quart) of cool water. The casualty should drink 3 to 5 canteenfuls during a period of 12 hours.

b. Heatstroke. Prolonged exposure to high temperature may cause heatstroke, which is sometimes referred to as "sunstroke." The first sign of heatstroke may be stoppage of sweating which causes the skin to feel hot and dry. Collapse and unconsciousness may come suddenly or may be preceded by headache, dizziness, fast pulse, nausea, vomiting, and mental confusion. It is necessary to work fast to save the life of a heatstroke casualty, as the heat regulators of the body have been damaged and the temperature may rise as high as 108° F. The following first aid measures should be administered promptly:

(1) Immerse the casualty in the coldest water available. If ice is available, add it to the water.

(2) If a cold water bath is not possible, get the casualty into the shade, remove his clothing, and keep his entire body wet by pouring water over him. Cool him further by continuously fanning his wet body.

(3) Transport him to the nearest medical treatment facility at once and continue to cool his body on the way.

(4) When the casualty becomes conscious, give him cool salt water to drink (*a*(2) above).

c. Heat Cramps. Heat cramps are painful spasms of the muscles, usually those of the legs, arms, and abdomen. They may be either mild or severe. Cramps are due directly to loss of salt from the body. Give a casualty with heat cramps large amounts of salt water to drink (*a*(2) above). If he has severe heat cramps, it may be necessary to send him to a medical treatment facility.

41. Conditions Caused by Cold

Conditions caused by cold are trench foot, immersion foot, frostbite, and snow blindness. These conditions can be prevented by practicing the prescribed preventive measures (FM 21–10).

a. Trench Foot. Trench foot is an injury which results from fairly long exposure of the feet to wet conditions, generally at temperatures from approximately freezing to 50° F. If the feet are also inactive, the possibility of developing trench foot is even greater. Trench foot can be very serious; it can lead to loss of toes or parts of the feet. Usually a symptom of trench foot is numbness. There may be a tingling or aching sensation or cramping pain. If exposure of the feet has been prolonged and severe, the feet may swell so tightly that pressure closes the blood vessels and cuts off the circulation. Should you develop trench foot, dry your feet thoroughly and get to a medical treatment facility by the shortest means possible. If transportation is available, avoid walking.

b. Immersion Foot. Immersion foot is similar to trench foot (*a* above) except in the manner in which it is caused. It results from immersion of the feet in water or constant wetness of the feet for a prolonged period, usually in excess of 12 hours. Immersion foot will develop more rapidly if the water is below 50° F. It can occur, however, when the feet are exposed even to warm water for a period exceeding 24 hours. In immersion foot the soles of the feet become wrinkled and white; standing or walking becomes extremely painful. Other portions of the body may be similarly affected. Should you develop immersion foot, dry your feet thoroughly and get to a medical treatment facility by the shortest means possible. If transportation is available, avoid walking.

c. Frostbite. Frostbite is the injury of tissue from exposure to cold. The body parts most easily frostbitten are the cheeks, nose, ears, chin, forehead, wrists, hands, and feet. Frostbite may involve only the skin, or it may extend to a depth below the skin. Deep frostbite, which is much more serious, requires different first aid to avoid or minimize the loss of the parts of the fingers, toes, hands, or feet. Frostbitten skin is whitish, stiff, and numb rather than painful. For this reason, soldiers must watch one another's face and hands for signs of frostbite. If the part has been numb for only a short time, the frostbite probably involves only the skin; otherwise assume it to be deep. The following measures should be taken for frostbite:

(1) *First aid measures for frostbite involving only the skin.*

Note. Do NOT warm or rewarm frostbitten parts by such measures as massage, exposure to open fire, cold water soaks, or rubbing with snow.

(*a*) *Parts of the face.* Cover the frostbitten part with your warm hands until pain returns.

(*b*) *Hands.* Place the bare hands next to the skin in the opposite armpits.

(*c*) *Feet.* In the most sheltered area available, place the bare feet under the clothing and against the abdomen of another soldier.

(2) *Measures to take when deep frostbite occurs.*

(*a*) Get to a medical treatment facility by the shortest means possible. If transportation is available, avoid walking.

(*b*) Protect the frostbitten part from additional injury, but do NOT attempt to treat it or thaw it in any way. Thawing in the field increases the possibilities of infection, further damage, and gangrene. There is less danger of walking on your feet while they are frozen than after they have been thawed. Thawing may occur spontaneously during transportation to the medical facility; but this cannot be avoided, as the body in general must be kept warm.

d. Snow Blindness. Snow blindness is the effect which glare from an icefield or snowfield has on the eyes. This condition can occur even in cloudy weather. In fact, it is more likely to occur in hazy, cloudy weather than when the sun is shining. The early stages of snow blindness can be recognized by the scratchy feeling in the eyes when the eyelids are closed. Should a person develop snow-blindness, his eyes should be covered with a dark cloth to shut out all light; then he should be taken to a medical treatment facility at once.

42. Carbon Monoxide (CO) Poisoning

a. Carbon monoxide poisoning can be severe, prolonged, and sometimes fatal. It results from inhaling carbon monoxide which is a colorless, tasteless, and practically odorless gas produced by the incomplete combustion of coal, oil, and other fuels used in such equipment as motor vehicles, field ranges, and lighting and heating devices. This carbon monoxide destroys the ability of the red blood cells to carry the needed oxygen to the body tissues. Carbon monoxide poisoning is usually the result of faulty equipment, improper use of equipment, or inadequate ventilation. It can be prevented by following the precautionary measures discussed in FM 21–10.

b. The symptoms of carbon monoxide poisoning come on rapidly and in quick succession. Dizziness, headache, noises in the ears, and throbbing in the temples are quickly followed by a feeling of sleepiness and weakness. Vomiting and convulsions may occur, followed by unconsciousness and death. The skin and lips are often bright red. The individual who is becoming poisoned may realize what is taking place, but he may not have enough strength left to get into the fresh air. Under circumstances in which there is muscular exertion or where there are extremes of temperature or humidity, the effects of poisoning act more rapidly.

c. The following first aid measures should be taken for a person who is overcome by carbon monoxide:

(1) Move the casualty into fresh air immediately and administer artificial respiration (para 8).

(2) Keep him quiet and transport him to a medical treatment facility.

43. Drowning

Drowning occurs when air is shut off from the airway by water or and other fluid, causing spasm of the vocal cords and blockage of the airway. Many casualties who appear lifeless may recover if artificial respiration (para 8) is performed promptly and efficiently. Speed is essential. Every moment of delay decreases the casualty's chance of survival. It is frequently possible to start the mouth-to-mouth method of artificial respiration (para 8*b*) before the casualty is brought ashore. As soon as his head is clear of the water and his mouth is within reach of your mouth, clear his airway and start artificial respiration. If other rescuers can help carry the casualty ashore, do not interrupt the artificial respiration. Once the casualty is ashored do not waste valuable seconds to turn him in an attempt to drain water from his lungs; but continue the artificial respiration.

44. Electrical Shock

Electric shock accidents frequently result from contact with a "live" wire and occasionally occur when a person is struck by lightning. If a person has come in contact with an electric current, take the following steps:

a. Turn off the switch if it is nearby, but do not waste time looking for it. Instead use a dry wooden pole, dry clothing, dry rope, or some other material which will not conduct electricity to remove the person from the wire. If a pole is not handy, simply drag the casualty off the wire by means of a loop of dry rope or cloth (fig 85). Do not touch the wire or the casualty with your bare hands or you will also get a shock.

b. Administer artificial respiration (para 8) immediately after

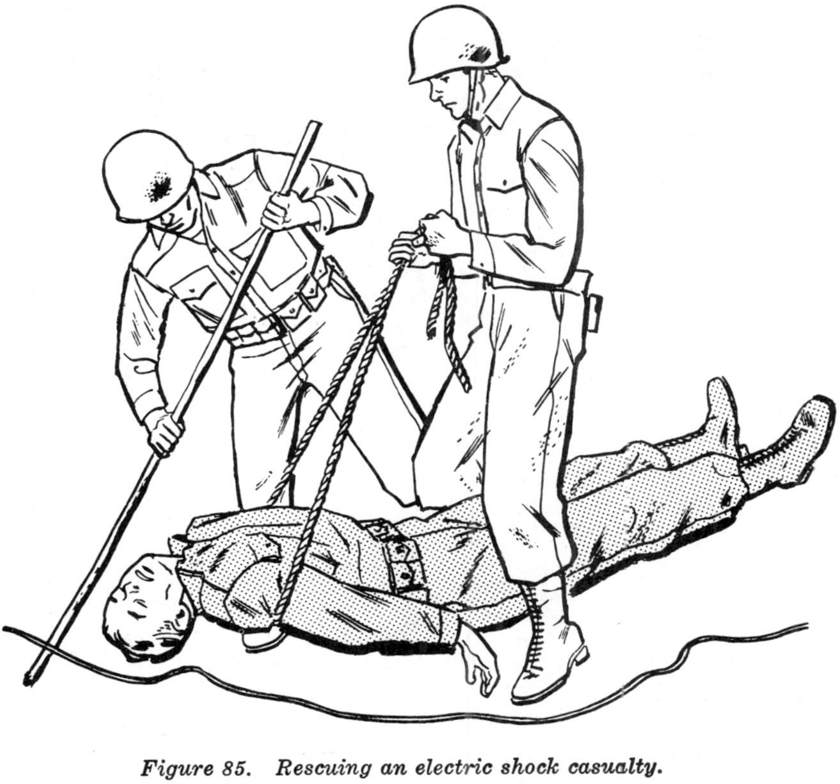

Figure 85. Rescuing an electric shock casualty.

freeing the person from the wire, as electric shock causes breathing to cease.

45. Unconsciousness

It is often impossible to find the cause of unconsciousness. Bleeding, heatstroke, or head injury may be the cause.

a. If a casualty is unconscious, apply the lifesaving measures A B C D (chap 2) as appropriate. If he has a head injury or a heatstroke, apply the special measures discussed in paragraph 21 or 40*b*. If the casualty remains unconscious after first aid measures have been applied, be sure to place him on his side or on his abdomen with his head turned to one side to prevent his choking on vomitus, blood, or other fluids (para 14*f*(2)). DO NOT give an unconscious casualty liquid.

b. If a casualty has merely fainted, he will regain consciousness in a few minutes. If an ammonia inhalant solution (app B) is available, break the ampul and place it near his nose several times for a few seconds each time. If he is in a sitting position, lay him down gently. Loosen his clothing, apply a cloth which has been wet with cool water to his face, and let him lie quietly. Anytime that a person is about to faint while sitting up, lower his head between his knees so that blood may flow to his head. Hold him so that he does not fall and injure himself.

CHAPTER 5

TRANSPORTATION OF SICK AND INJURED

46. General

a. Knowing how to transport a seriously injured casualty is one of the most important parts of first aid. Careless or rough handling not only may increase the seriousness of his injury but also may cause his death. Unless there is a good reason for transporting a casualty, do not do so until some means of medical evacuation is provided. Sometimes when the situation is urgent and you know that no medical evacuation facilities are available, you will have to transport the casualty yourself. That is why you should know the

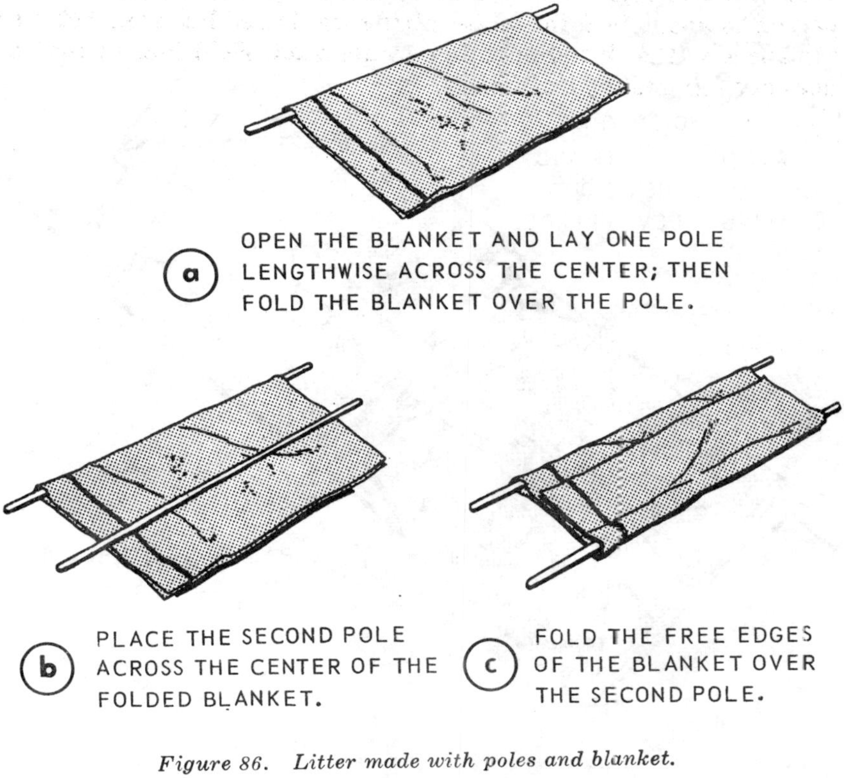

Figure 86. Litter made with poles and blanket.

different ways of transporting a casualty. Give the casualty the appropriate first aid before leaving with him. If he has a broken bone, do not transport him until you have splinted or immobilized the part.

b. This chapter describes ways of improvising a litter and methods of carrying a casualty without a litter. Do not transport a casualty with a fractured back or neck without a litter. If the casualty has a fracture of any other part, transport him in a way which will not aggravate the fracture. An unconscious casualty should be transported on a litter or carried in such a way that he will not fall. Transportation by litter is safer and more comforta-

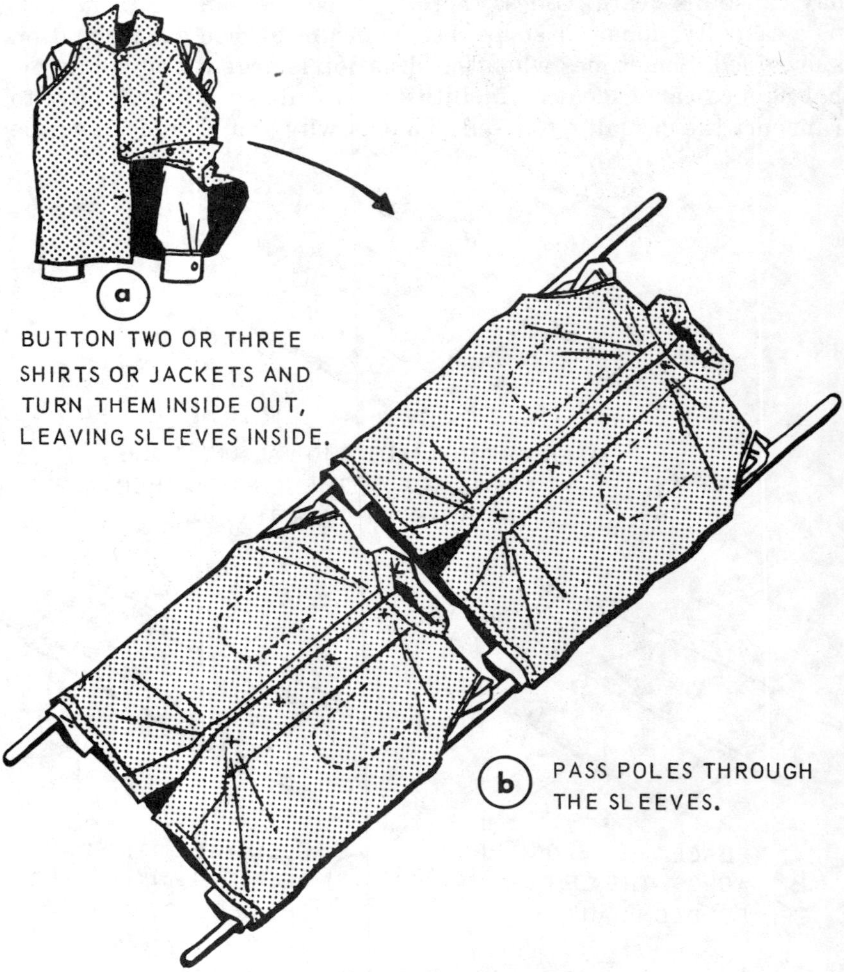

Figure 87. Litter made with poles and jackets.

ble for all casualties as well as easier for you. If carrying the casualty is the only feasible method because of the terrain or the combat situation or is necessary to save the casualty's life, it should be used; but the casualty should be transferred to a litter as soon as one can be made available or improvised.

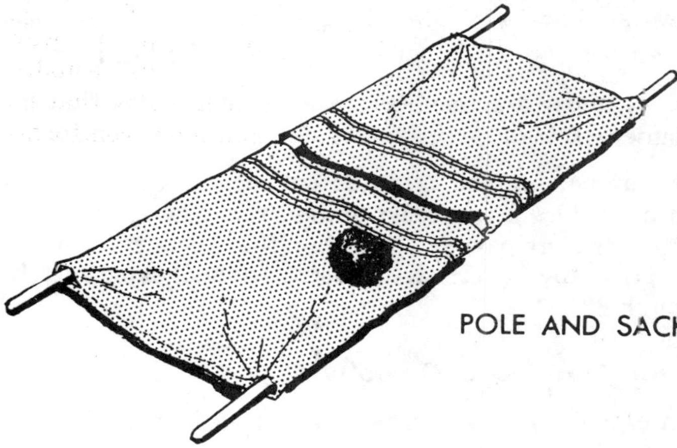

POLE AND SACK LITTER

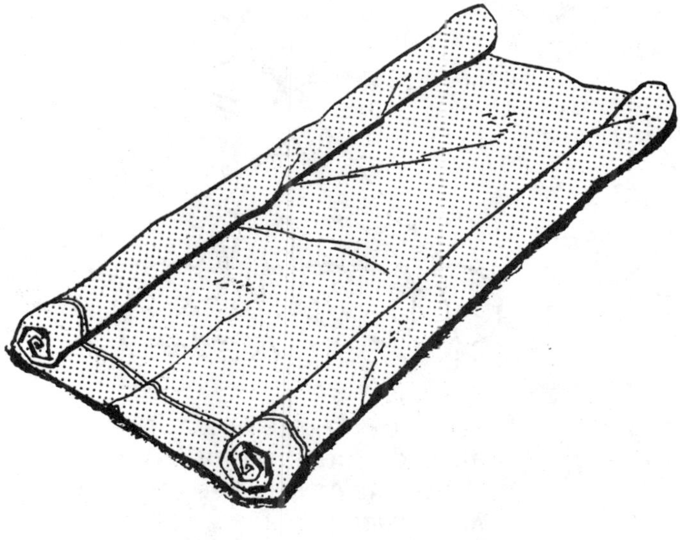

BLANKET ROLL LITTER

Figure 88. Litters made by inserting poles through sacks and by rolling blanket.

7. Improvised Litters

a. A litter can be improvised from many different things. Most flat-surface objects of suitable size can be used as litters. Such objects include boards, doors, window shutters, benches, ladders, cots, and poles tied together. If possible, such objects should be padded.

b. Satisfactory litters can be also made by securing poles inside such items as blankets, shelter halves, tarpaulins, jackets, shirts, sacks, bags, bedticks, and mattress covers. Poles can be improvised from strong branches, rifles, tent supports, skis, and other items.

Caution: **If weapons are used as splints, be absolutely sure they are unloaded.**

c. If no poles can be obtained, a large item such as a blanket can be rolled from both sides toward the center; then the rolls can be used to obtain a firm grip when carrying the casualty. Several methods of improvising litters are illustrated and explained in figures 86 through 88.

48. Methods of Carrying a Casualty

a. General. A casualty may be transported by using one-man and

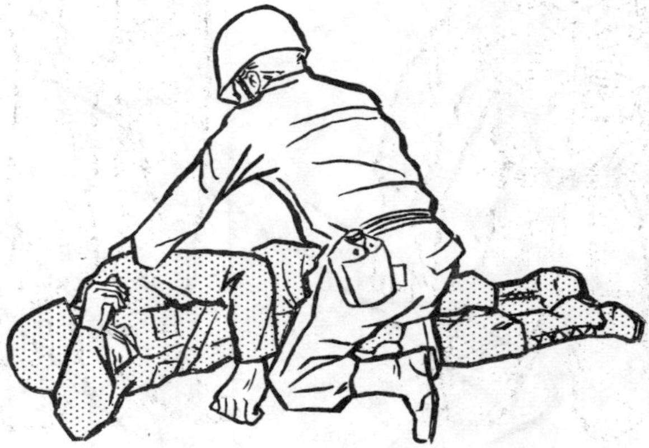

STEP ONE: IF THE CASUALTY IS LYING ON HIS BACK, KNEEL AT HIS UNINJURED SIDE, PLACE ONE OF HIS ARMS ACROSS HIS FACE, AND GENTLY ROLL HIM TOWARD YOU ONTO HIS ABDOMEN. HIS ARM PROTECTS HIS FACE FROM THE GROUND.

Figure 89①. Fireman's carry (step one).

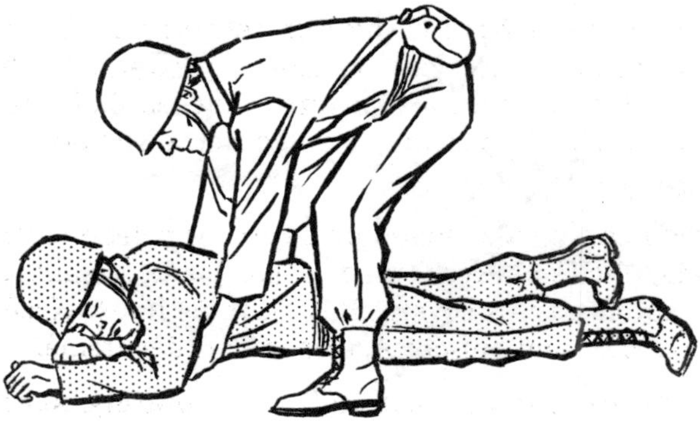

STEP TWO: STRADDLE THE CASUALTY AND GRASP HIM BY EXTENDING YOUR HANDS UNDER HIS ARMPITS AND AGAINST HIS CHEST.

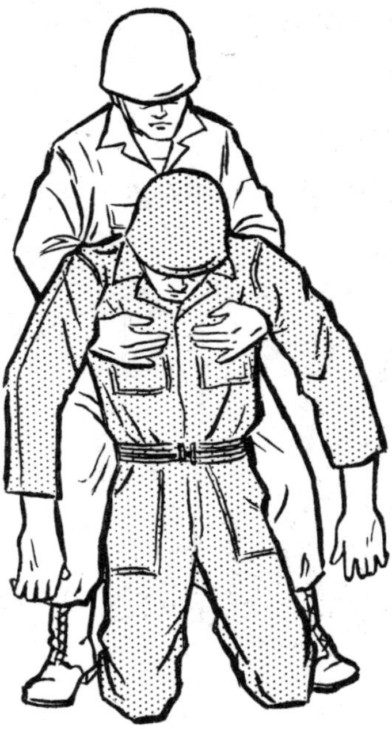

STEP THREE: LIFT THE CASUALTY TO HIS KNEES; THEN SECURE YOUR HOLD AND RAISE HIM TO A STANDING POSITION UNTIL HIS KNEES LOCK.

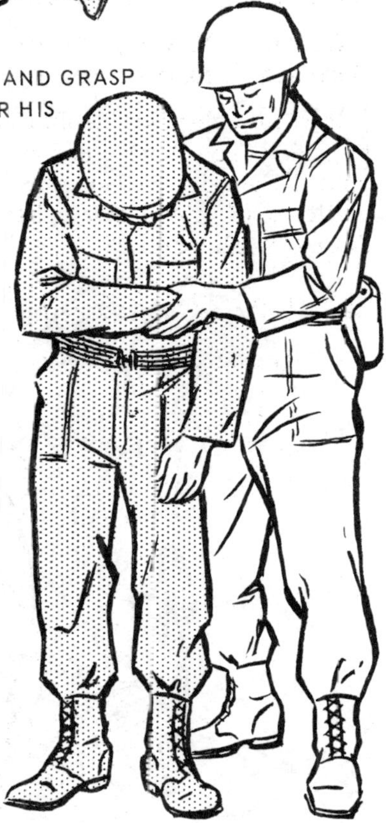

STEP FOUR: SUPPORTING THE CASUALTY WITH YOUR RIGHT ARM AROUND HIS WAIST, TAKE HOLD OF HIS RIGHT WRIST WITH YOUR LEFT HAND AND MOVE IN FRONT OF HIM.

Figure 89②. Fireman's carry (steps two, three, and four).

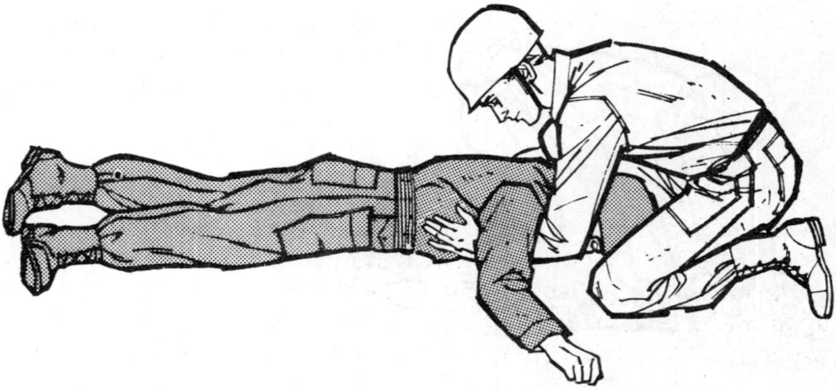

STEP TWO: KNEEL ON ONE KNEE AT THE CASUALTY'S HEAD, FACING HIS FEET; THEN GRASP HIM BY EXTENDING YOUR HANDS UNDER HIS ARMPITS, DOWN HIS SIDES, AND ACROSS HIS BACK.

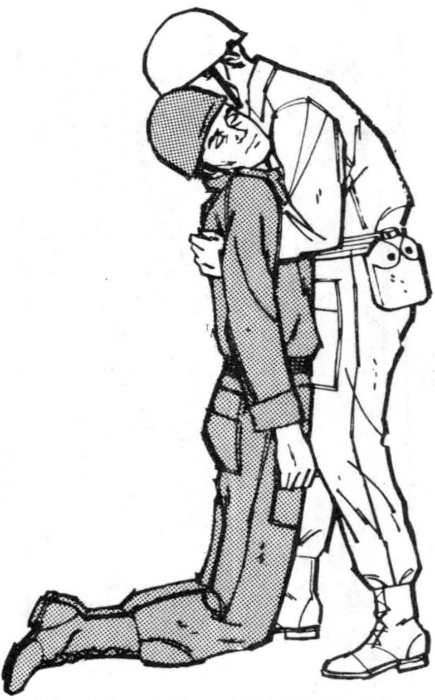

STEP THREE: AS YOU RISE, LIFT THE CASUALTY TO HIS KNEES; THEN SECURE YOUR HOLD AND RAISE HIM TO A STANDING POSITION UNTIL HIS KNEES LOCK.

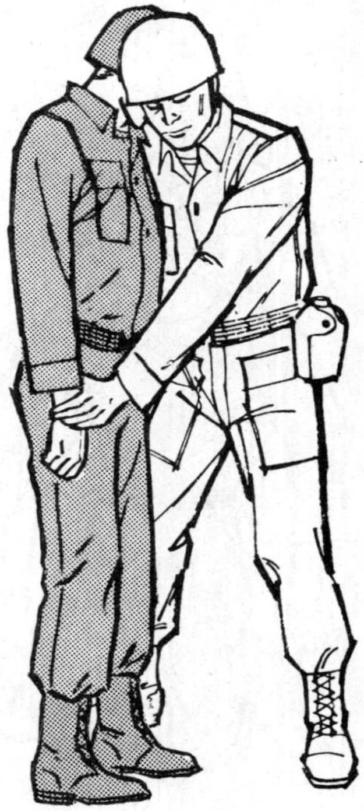

STEP FOUR: SUPPORTING THE CASUALTY WITH YOUR RIGHT ARM AROUND HIS WAIST, TAKE HOLD OF HIS RIGHT WRIST WITH YOUR LEFT HAND.

Figure 89③. Fireman's carry (steps two, three and four alternate method).

two-man carries. The two-man carries should be used whenever possible, as they provide more comfort to the casualty, are less likely to aggravate his injury, and are less tiring to the carriers. The particular one-man or two-man carry selected for use should be the one which is least likely to aggravate the casualty's injury.

b. Fireman's Carry. This method is one of the easiest ways for one man to get a casualty off the ground and to carry him (1–5, fig 89). The steps (two, three, and four) for getting the casualty off the ground may be accomplished in one of two ways, depending upon the location of the casualty's injury. The carrier should decide which method would be better for the casualty. Furthermore, the

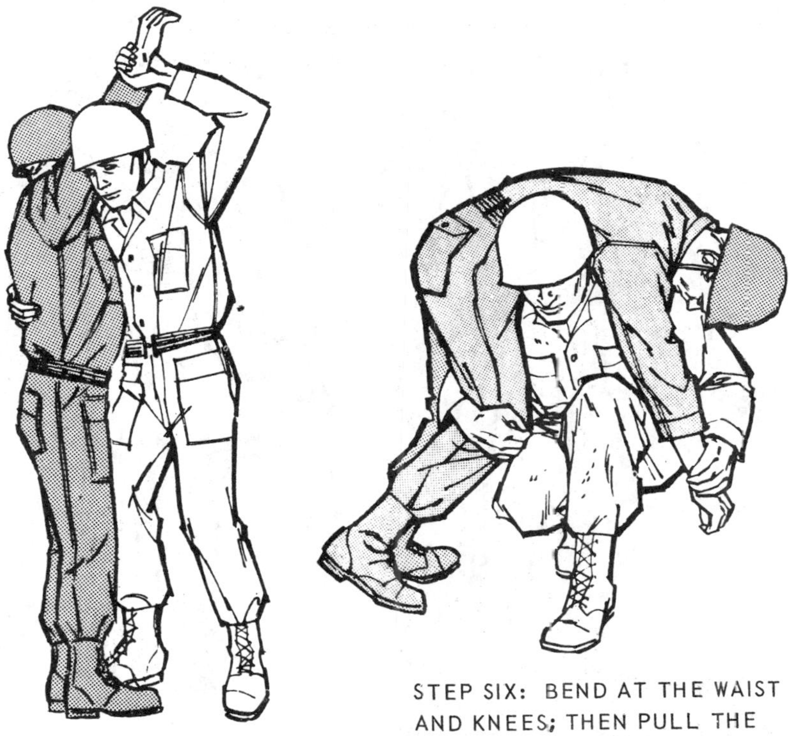
STEP FIVE: RAISE THE CASUALTY'S RIGHT ARM OVER YOUR HEAD.
STEP SIX: BEND AT THE WAIST AND KNEES; THEN PULL THE CASUALTY'S ARM OVER AND DOWN YOUR LEFT SHOULDER, THUS BRINGING HIS BODY ACROSS YOUR SHOULDERS. AT THE SAME TIME PASS YOUR RIGHT ARM BETWEEN HIS LEGS AND GRASP HIS RIGHT KNEE WITH YOUR HAND.

Figure 89(4). Fireman's carry (steps five and six).

carrier should bring the casualty onto his back from the side which will avoid pressure on the injured part.

c. Supporting Carry. This carry is useful when the casualty is only slightly injured.

(1) Lift the casualty off the ground as illustrated in the first three steps of the fireman's carry (1, 2 and 3, fig 89).

(2) Grasp the wrist of the casualty's uninjured arm and draw his arm around your neck (fig 90).

(3) Let the casualty walk, using you as a crutch.

d. Arms Carry. This carry is useful for a short distance.

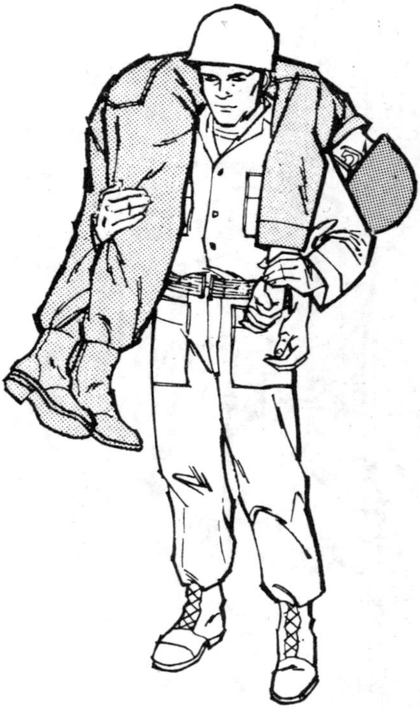

STEP SEVEN: STAND WITH CASUALTY ON YOUR SHOULDERS.

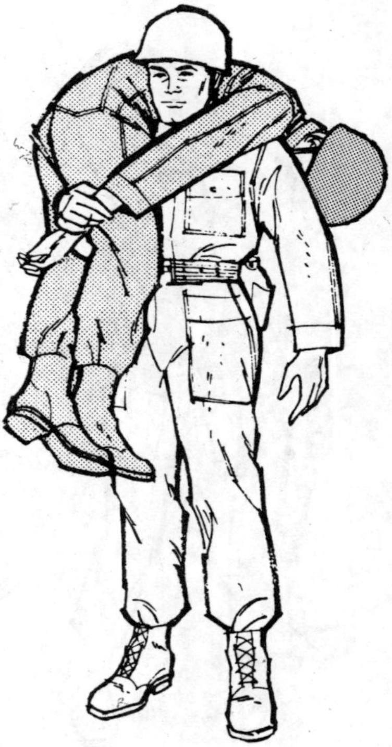

STEP EIGHT: GRASP THE CASUALTY'S RIGHT WRIST WITH YOUR RIGHT HAND, LEAVING YOUR LEFT HAND FREE. A MAN CAN CARRY ANOTHER PERSON SOME DISTANCE IN THIS MANNER.

Figure 89(5). Fireman's carry (steps seven and eight).

(1) Lift the casualty off the ground as illustrated in the first three steps of the fireman's carry (l, 2 or 3 fig 89).

(2) Position your arms on the casualty as illustrated in figure 91 and lift him into your arms.

(3) Carry the casualty high to lessen fatigue.

e. Saddleback Carry.

(1) Lift the casualty off the ground as illustrated in the first three steps of the fireman's carry (1, 2 or 3, fig 89).

(2) Supporting the casualty with one of your arms around him, turn so that the casualty can encircle your neck with his arms;

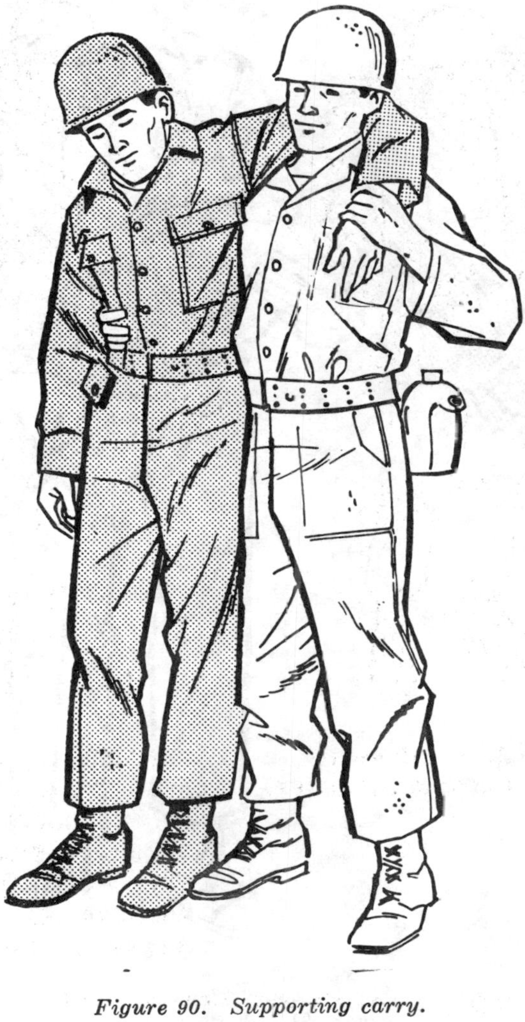

Figure 90. Supporting carry.

then stoop, clasp your hands beneath his thighs, and raise him upon your back (fig 92).

f. Pack-Strap Carry.

(1) Lift the casualty off the ground as illustrated in the first three steps of the fireman's carry (1, 2 or 3, fig 89).

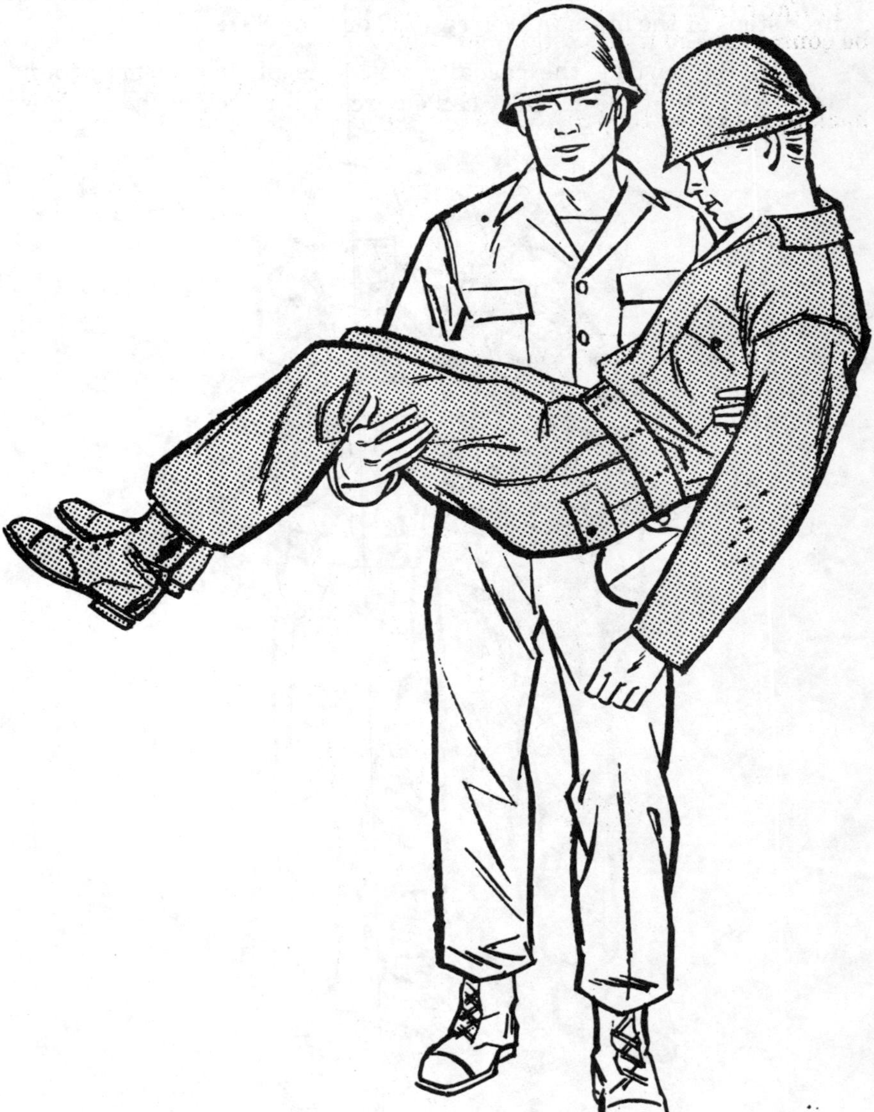

Figure 91. Arms carry.

(2) Supporting the casualty with your arm around him, grasp his wrist which is closest to you and place his arm over your head and across your shoulders; then move in front of him while supporting his weight against your back, grasp his other wrist, and place this arm over your shoulder (a, fig 93).

(3) Bend forward and hoist him as high on your back as possible so that all his weight is resting on your back (b, fig 93).

g. Back Lift and Carry. For use of this carry, the casualty must be conscious and able to stand on at least one leg.

(1) Raise the casualty to a standing position and place your back to his back; then have him stretch out his arms sideways.

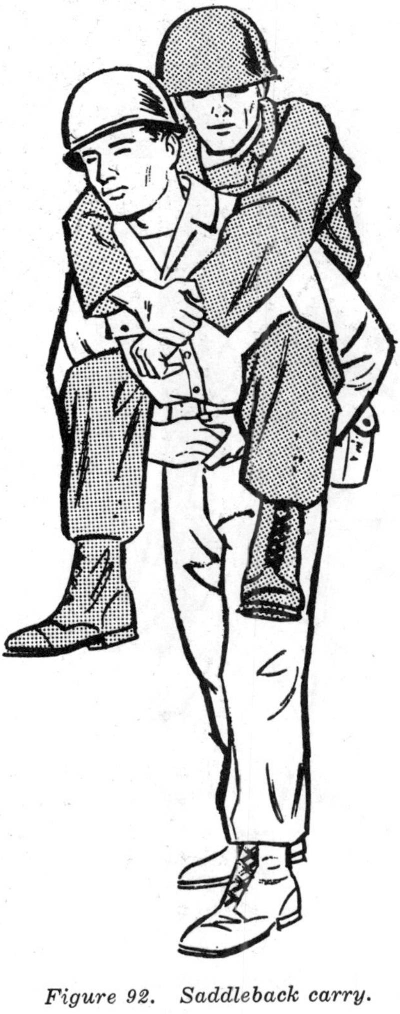

Figure 92. Saddleback carry.

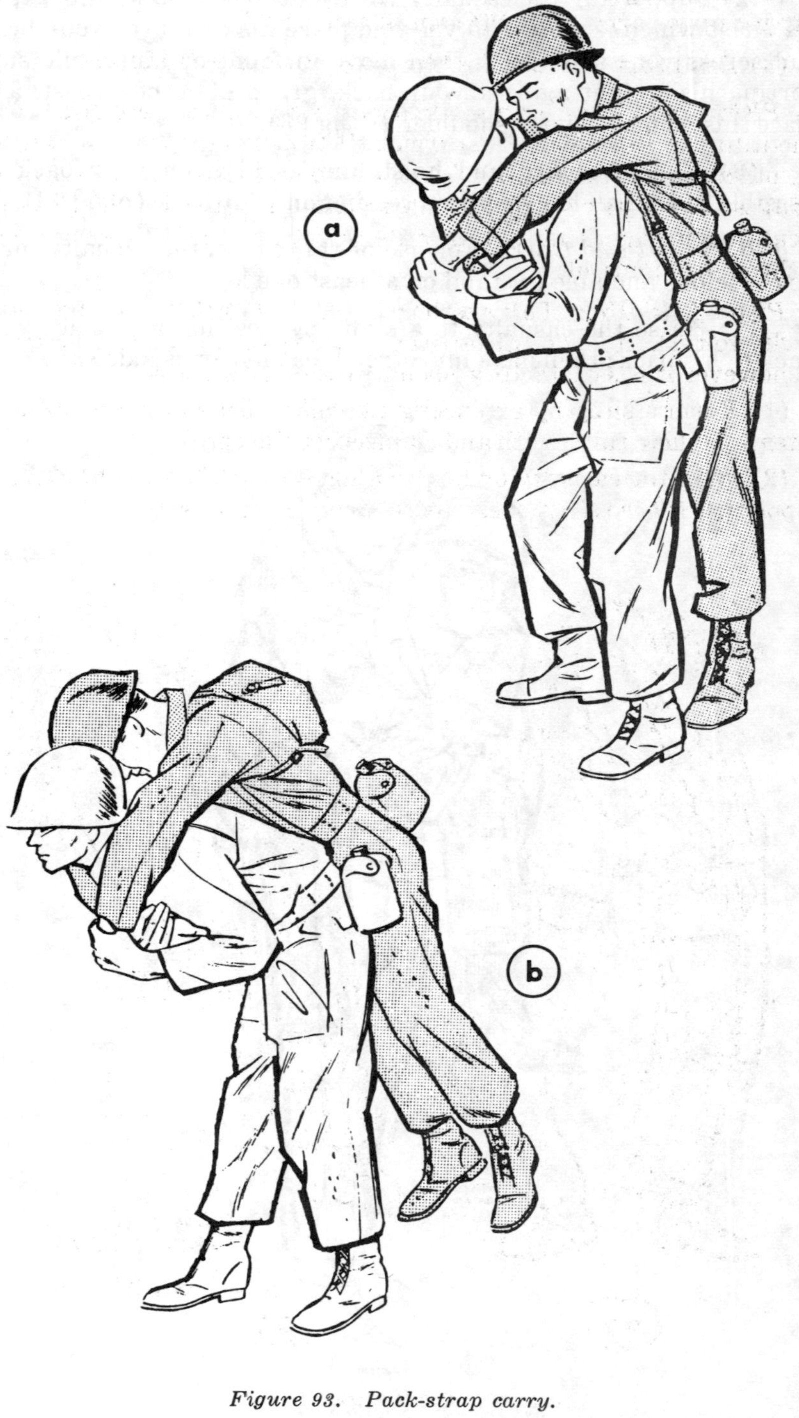

Figure 93. Pack-strap carry.

(2) Bending backward, put your hands under his arms and grasp his upper arms near the armpits (a, fig 94).

(3) Bend forward, pulling him onto your back (b, fig 94).

h. Pistol-Belt Carry. This method can be used for a long distance without undue fatigue on the carrier. If pistol belts are not available, other items can be used, such as one rifle sling, two cravat bandages, two litter straps, or any suitable material which will not cut or bind the casualty. The steps in this method are provided in 1 through 3 figure 95.

i. Pistol-Belt Drag. This method (fig. 96) enables you and the casualty to remain low on the ground, more protected from enemy fire; however it is satisfactory for only a short distance.

(1) Form a sling by extending two pistol belts or other suitable items to their full length and connecting the ends.

(2) With the casualty on his back, pass the sling over his head and position it across his chest and under his armpits.

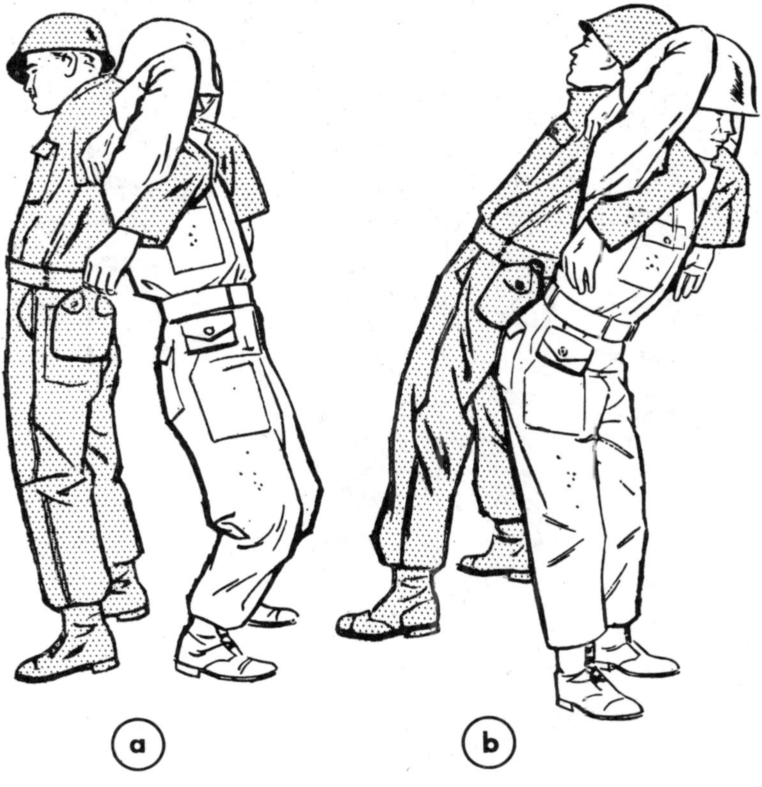

Figure 94. Back lift and carry.

(3) Cross the sling straps at a point near the casualty's shoulder, forming a loop for your shoulder.

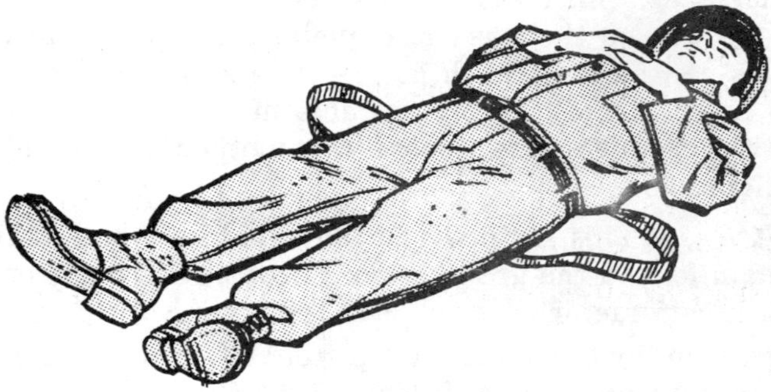

STEP ONE: LINK TOGETHER TWO PISTOL BELTS TO FORM A SLING. PLACE THE SLING UNDER THE CASUALTY'S THIGHS AND LOWER BACK SO THAT A LOOP EXTENDS FROM EACH SIDE.

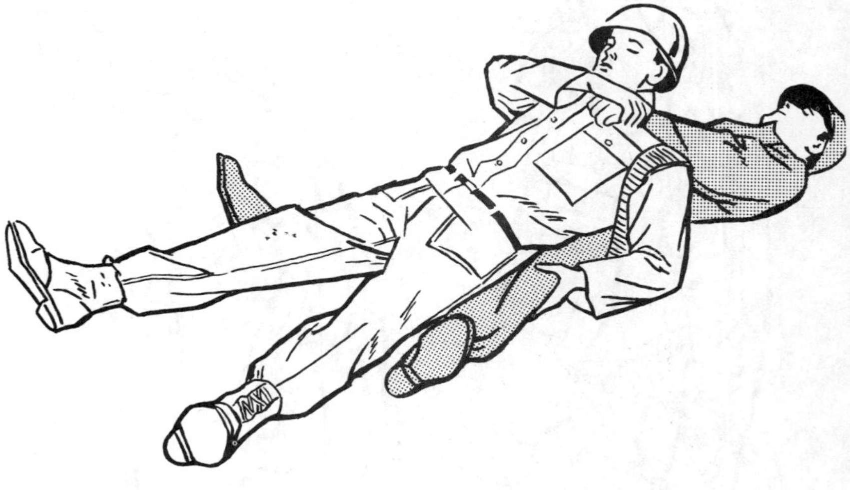

STEP TWO: LIE BETWEEN THE CASUALTY'S OUTSTRETCHED LEGS. THRUST YOUR ARMS THROUGH THE LOOPS. GRASP CASUALTY'S HAND AND TROUSER LEG ON HIS INJURED SIDE.

Figure 95(1). Pistol-belt carry (steps one and two).

(4) Lie on your back beside the casualty and slip the loop over your arm which is closer to the casualty; then turn away from the casualty onto your abdomen, thus causing the loop to fit tightly around your shoulder.

(5) Place your arm which is nearer the casualty underneath his head to protect it during movement.

(6) Crawl along, dragging the casualty with you.

j. Neck Drag. This method (fig 97) enables you and the casualty to remain close to the ground.

(1) Tie the casualty's hands together and loop them around your neck.

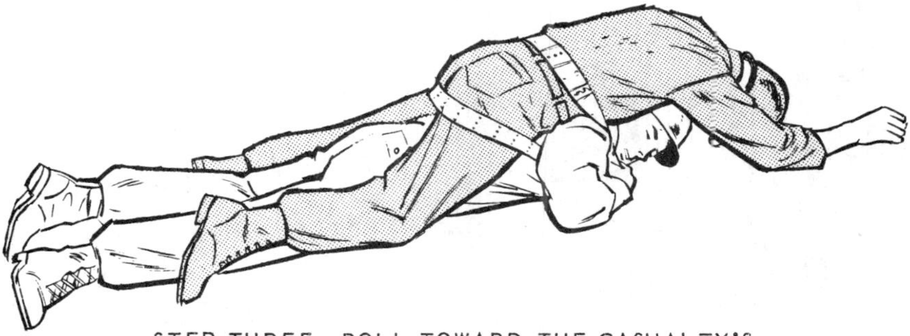

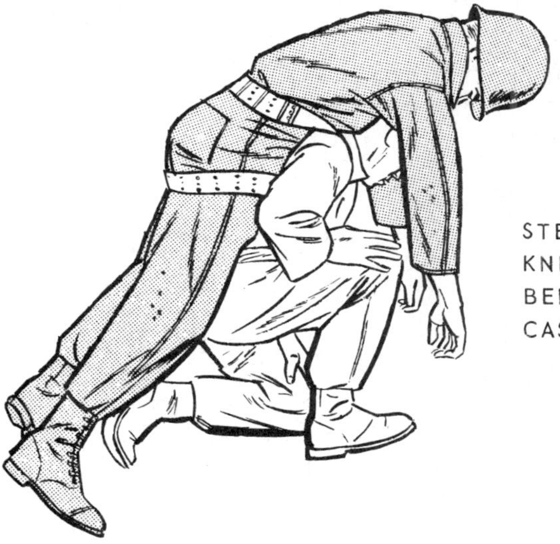

Figure 95②. Pistol-belt carry (steps three and four).

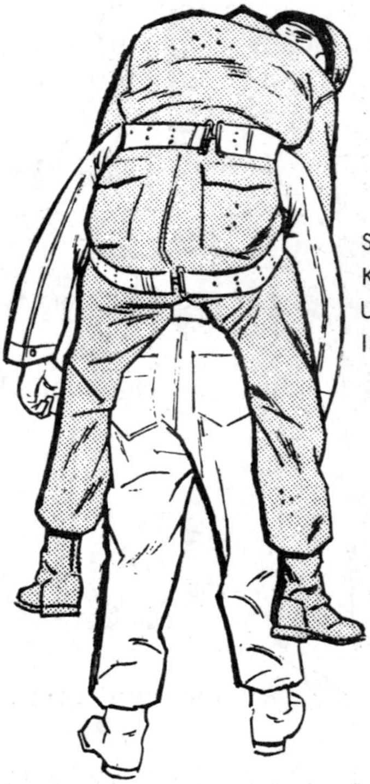

STEP FIVE: PLACE ONE HAND ON YOUR KNEE FOR SUPPORT AND RISE TO AN UPRIGHT POSITION. THE CASUALTY IS NOW SUPPORTED ON YOUR SHOULDERS.

STEP SIX: CARRY THE CASUALTY WITH YOUR HANDS FREE FOR USE IN FIRING RIFLE, CLIMBING BANKS, OR SURMOUNTING OBSTACLES.

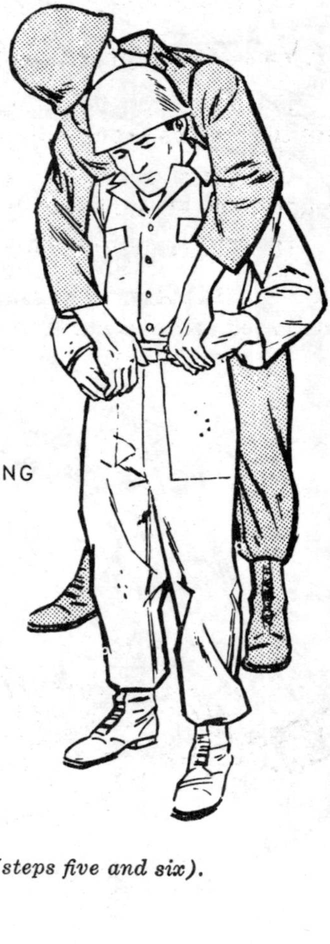

Figure 95③. Pistol-belt carry (steps five and six).

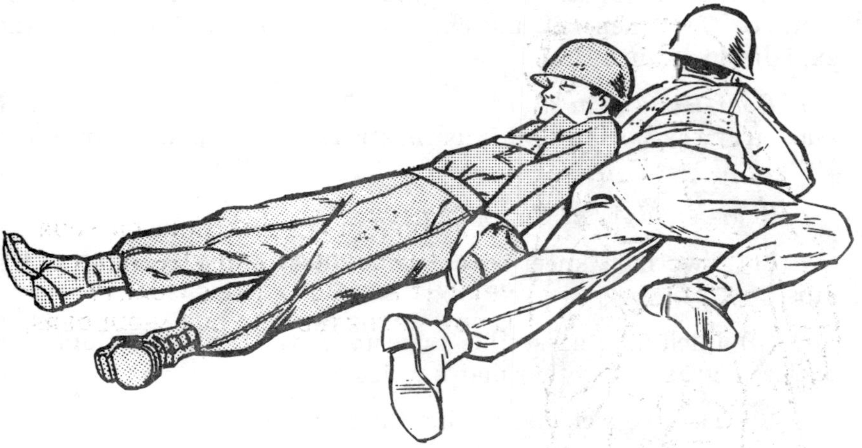

Figure 96. Pistol-belt drag.

(2) Crawl along, dragging the casualty with you.

k. Two-Man Supporting Carry (fig 98).

(1) Two men help the casualty to his feet and support him with their arms around his waist.

(2) They grasp the casualty's wrists and draw his arms around their necks.

(3) The casualty walks, using the two men as crutches.

l. Two-Man Arms Carry. Two men lift and carry the casualty as illustrated and explained in figure 99.

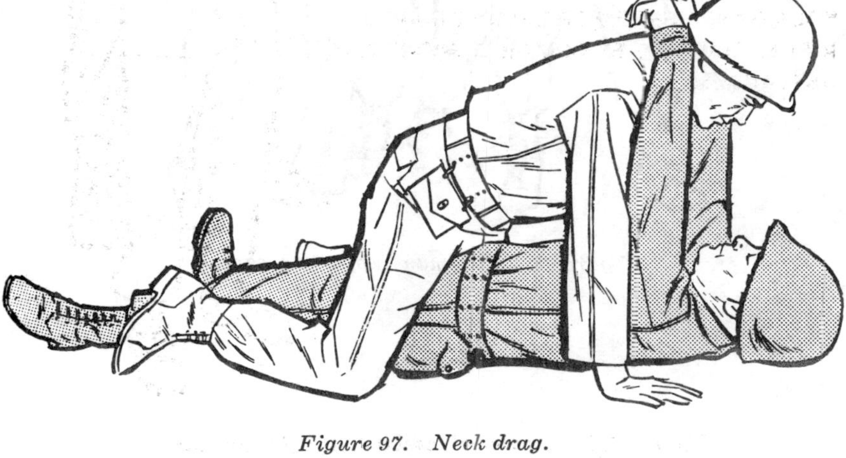

Figure 97. Neck drag.

m. Two-Man Saddleback Carry. This carry is useful for a short distance. Two men lift and carry the casualty as illustrated and explained in figure 100.

n. Four-Hand (Packsaddle) Carry. Two men make a packsaddle and carry the casualty on it as illustrated and explained in figure 101.

o. Four-Hand Arms Carry (fig 102).

(1) Two men kneel on opposite sides of the casualty at his hips.

(2) Each man passes his arms under the casualty's thigh and back and grasps the other man's wrist.

(3) The two men rise, lifting the casualty.

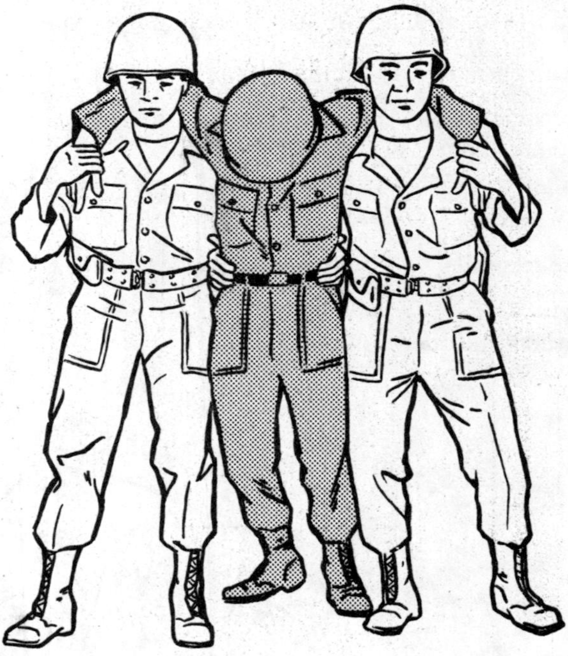

Figure 98. Two-man supporting carry.

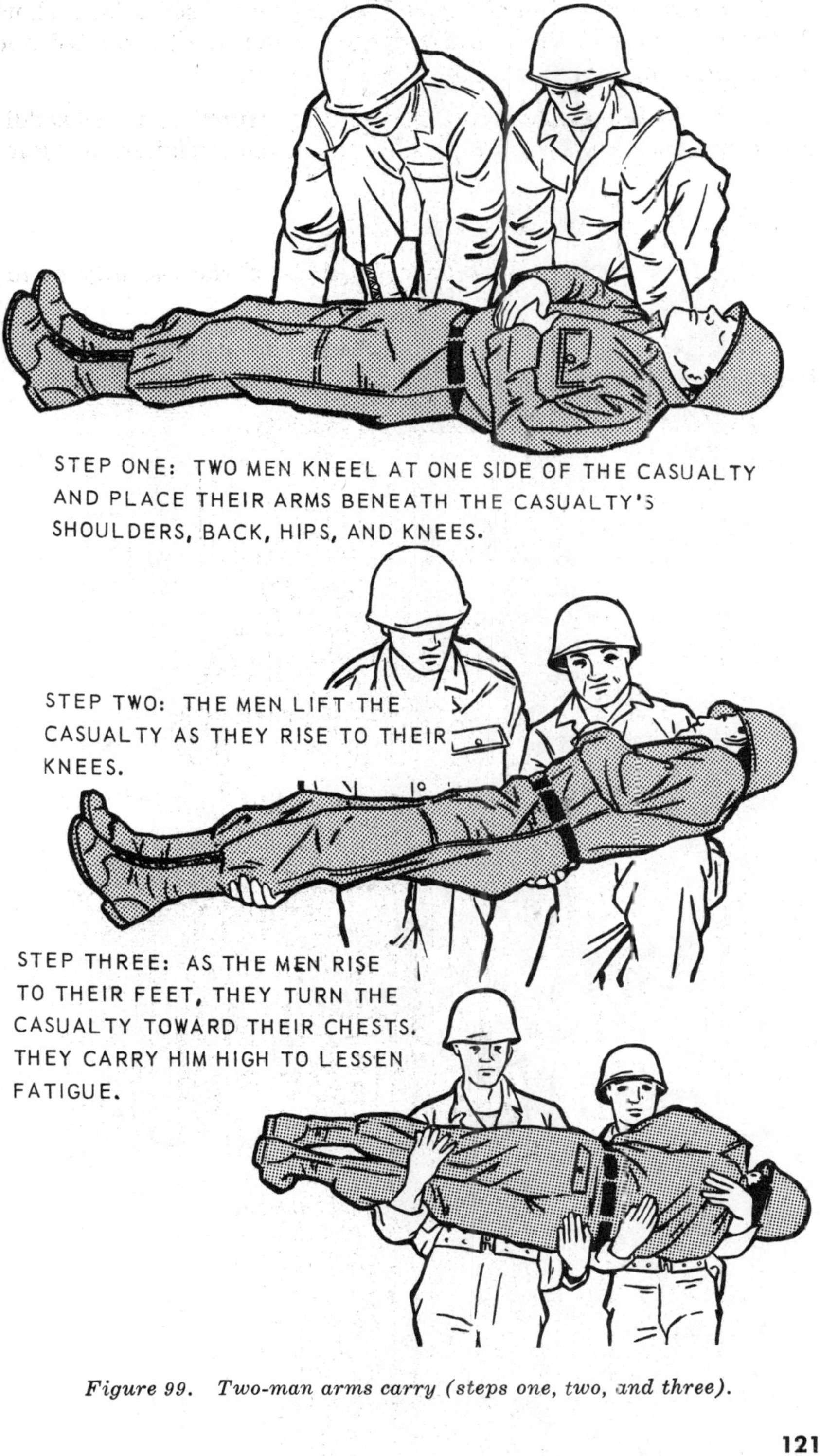

Figure 99. Two-man arms carry (steps one, two, and three).

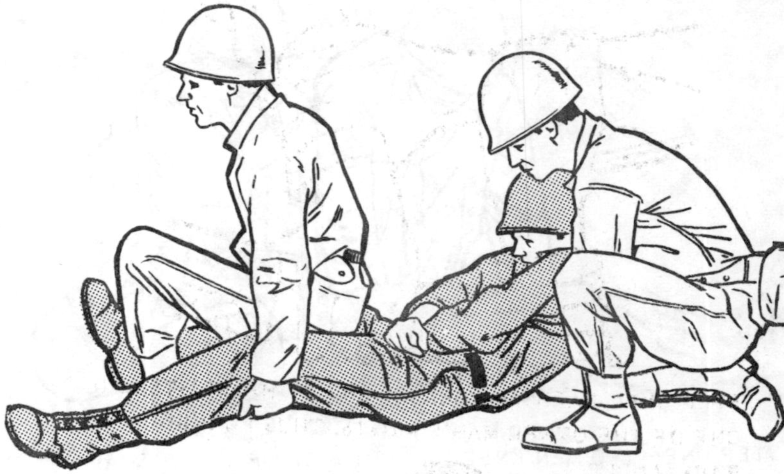

STEP ONE: ONE MAN SPREADS THE CASUALTY'S LEGS, KNEELS BETWEEN THE LEGS WITH HIS BACK TO THE CASUALTY, AND POSITIONS HIS HANDS BEHIND THE KNEES. THE OTHER MAN KNEELS AT THE CASUALTY'S HEAD, SLIDES HIS HANDS UNDER THE ARMS AND ACROSS THE CHEST, AND LOCKS HIS HANDS TOGETHER.

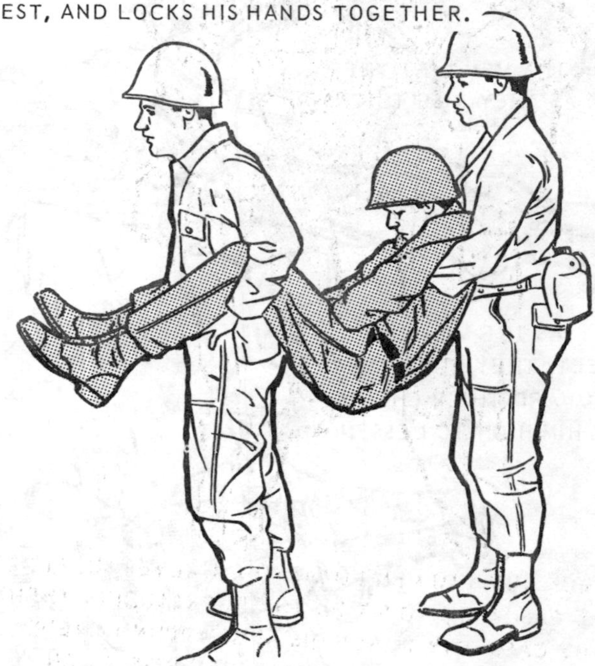

STEP TWO: THE TWO MEN RISE TOGETHER, LIFTING THE CASUALTY.

Figure 100. Two-man saddleback carry (steps one and two).

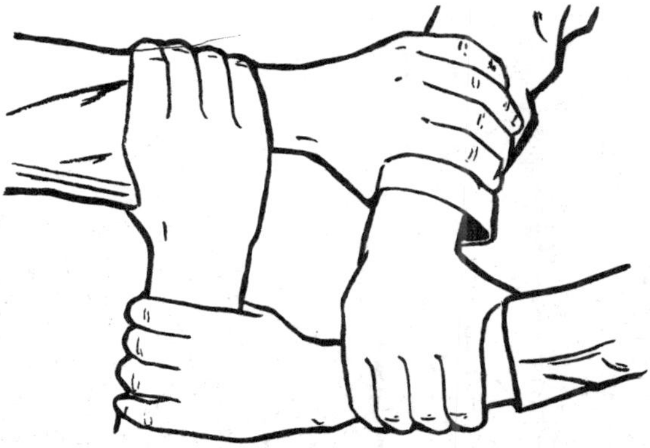

STEP ONE: EACH MAN GRASPS ONE OF HIS WRISTS AND ONE OF THE OTHER MAN'S WRISTS, THUS FORMING A PACKSADDLE.

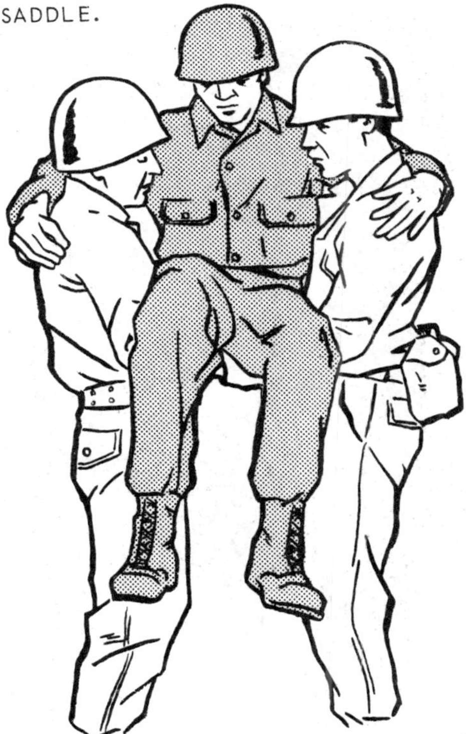

STEP TWO: THE TWO MEN LOWER THEMSELVES SUFFICIENTLY FOR THE CASUALTY TO SIT ON THE PACKSADDLE; THEN THEY HAVE THE CASUALTY PLACE HIS ARMS AROUND THEIR SHOULDERS FOR SUPPORT BEFORE THEY RISE TO AN UPRIGHT POSITION.

Figure 101. Four-hand (packsaddle) carry (steps one and two).

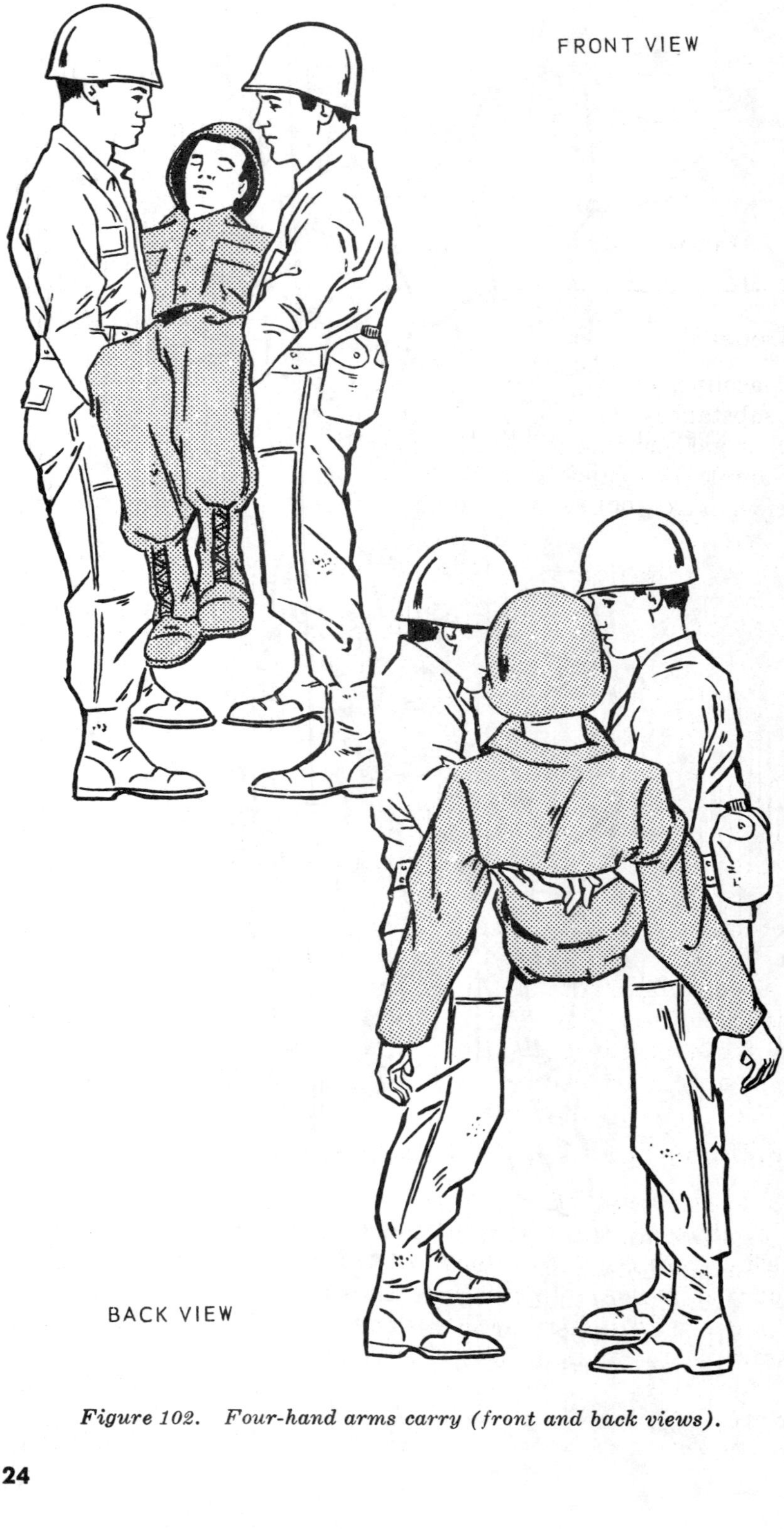

Figure 102. Four-hand arms carry (front and back views).

CHAPTER 6

FIRST AID IN A TOXIC ENVIRONMENT

49. General

a. Gasoline, chlorine, and pesticides are examples of common toxic substances. They may exist in the physical state as a solid, liquid, or gas, depending upon temperature and pressure. Gasoline, for example, is a vaporizable liquid; chlorine is a gas; and DDT, a pesticide, is a solid. Some substances are more injurious to the body than others when they are inhaled, are eaten, or come in contact with body surfaces. Whether they are solids, liquids, or gases (vapors and aerosols included), they may irritate, inflame, burn, freeze, or destroy tissue such as that associated with the respiratory tract or the eyes. They may also be absorbed into the blood stream, thus causing disturbance to any one of the body's major functions.

b. You may come in contact with toxic substances in everyday use such as the use of disinfectants and of bleach solutions for cleaning clothes, through accidents in handling chemicals, or through exposure to chemical agents used as a means of warfare. Ordinarily, exposure to a toxic substance would be for only a period of minutes; however in warfare any toxic substance employed by the enemy would be such that it could persist for hours or days. This would produce a toxic environment in which you would have to live. You must, therefore, be prepared to protect yourself and others against the injurious effects of these agents and to give first aid, when necessary, within this toxic environment.

50. Protective and First Aid Equipment

You are issued equipment for protection against field concentrations of chemical and biological agents. Such equipment includes the field protective mask, automatic atropine injectors, and absorptive powder for decontamination of your skin and clothing. You must know when and how to use these items. When considered necessary, you will also be issued special protective clothing, "dubbing" for boots (vesicant agent resistant leather dressing), and other prophylactic and/or first aid drugs as required.

a. Field Protective Mask (Model ABC–M17 or M17A1). Your field protective mask is a *most important* piece of protective equipment. You are given special training in its use and care. If you are equipped with the M17A1 protective mask, see paragraph 25*b*(2)(*c*) for explanation of the drinking tube and the protective canteen cap.

b. Automatic Atropine Injectors. You are issued for your own use three automatic atropine injectors, each containing 2 milligrams of the drug. The injectors are individually sealed in plastic. They are to be carried in the upper outer pocket of your field protective mask carrier.

c. M13 Individual Decontaminating and Reimpregnating Kit. This kit which is effective against chemical agents consists of—

(1) One skin decontaminating pad for use in absorbing droplets of chemical agents from your skin. It is a continuous belt-type pad designed to fit over your gloved fingers.

(2) Two bags, each containing chloramide powder and a dye capsule for use in neutralizing and indicating droplets of liquid chemical agents on your clothing and personal equipment as described in FM 21–41.

(3) A cutter to remove from your clothing the contaminated areas indicated by the dye ((2) above).

Note. The contents of this kit should NOT be used in or around the eyes. Only water should be used to flush chemical agents from the eyes.

51. Protective and First Aid Measures for Chemical-Biological Agents

a. General.

(1) Chemical agents for warfare uses may be classified according to the primary physiological effects they produce, such as nerve, blister, blood, choking, vomiting, and tear (lacrimators) agents. Your field protective mask gives protection against chemical agents as well as biological agents and the breathing in of radioactive particles. By means of previous practice, you should be able to mask in 9 seconds or less.

(2) Ingesting water or food contaminated with nerve, blister, and other chemical agents and some biological agents can be fatal. Never consume water or food which could have become contaminated until it has been tested and found safe for consumption.

b. Conditions For Masking Without Order Or Alarm. Once an attack with a chemical or biological agent is detected or suspected or information is available that such an agent is about to be used, you must mask immediately and not wait to receive an order or alarm when—

(1) Your position is hit by—

(*a*) Artillery or mortor fire.

(*b*) Missiles or rockets.

(*c*) Smoke or mists.

(*d*) Aerial spray or bombs.

(2) Smoke from an unknown source is present.

(3) A suspicious odor, liquid, or solid is present.

(4) You are entering an area suspected of being contaminated.

(5) You have one or more of the following symptoms:

(*a*) An unexplained runny nose.

(*b*) A feeling of choking or tightness in the chest or throat.

(*c*) Dimming of vision.

(*d*) Irritation of the eyes.

(*e*) Difficulty in or increased rates of breathing without obvious reasons.

c. First Aid Steps For A Chemical Attack.

(1) *Step ONE.* Stop breathing, put on your mask and clear it, give the alarm, and continue mission.

Note. Keep your mask on until it has been determined that the area is no longer hazardous and you are told to unmask.

(2) *Step TWO.* If symptoms of nerve agent poisoning (para 52*b*) appear, give yourself an atropine injection (para 52*c*).

Note. Do NOT inject atropine until you are sure that it is needed.

(3) *Step THREE.* If you suspect chemical agent droplets in your eyes, accomplish the following actions as rapidly as possible. To be effective against mustard agents (para 53), they must be accomplished within 2 minutes.

(*a*) Unscrew the cap on your canteen.

(*b*) Remove your helmet.

(*c*) Take and hold a deep breath and raise your mask so that your face is uncovered.

(*d*) To flush your right eye, tilt your head back and slightly to the right. To flush your left eye, tilt your head back and slightly to the left.

(*e*) With your eyes looking upward, pour water into your

eye slowly, if possible, so that the water will not run onto your face and clothing. If you cannot keep your eye open, pull your eyelids away from your eye with your fingers.

(*f*) Reseat and clear your mask.

(4) *Step FOUR.* If you suspect that your face is contaminated, accomplish the following actions:

(*a*) Take your M13 kit (para 50*c*) from your protective mask carrier and open it.

(*b*) Take the skin decontaminating pad from the M13 kit and insert it over your gloved fingers.

(*c*) Take and hold a deep breath and raise your mask so that your face is uncovered.

(*d*) Blot the liquid contamination from your face with the skin decontaminating pad.

(*e*) Rotate the skin decontaminating pad and slap it on your face to release the powder; then rub the powder over the contaminated areas of your face. Do NOT get the powder in your eyes.

(*f*) If you suspect that a chemical agent is inside your mask, use the skin decontaminating pad to decontaminate the inside, applying the same techniques described in *d* and *e* above.

(*g*) Reseat and clear your mask.

(5) *Step FIVE.* As soon as your mission permits, remove any liquid contamination from other skin areas with the skin decontaminating pad from your M13 kit, using the same technique described in (4)(*d*) and (*e*) above.

(6) *Step SIX.* If nerve agents are used and your mission permits, be on the lookout for persons who need additional atropine injections and administer them.

(7) *Step SEVEN.* When your mission permits, decontaminate your personal clothing and equipment, using the bags of chloramide powder and cutter from your M13 kit as described in FM 21–41.

52. Nerve Agents

a. General. Nerve agents may enter the body through the eyes and the skin and by breathing and eating. Although the nerve agents can be absorbed into the body through unbroken skin, they do not produce a localized irritant effect. Smoking is not permitted for at least 24 hours after exposure to a nerve agent, as the tars and nicotine will increase and prolong the nerve agent effects.

b. Symptoms of Nerve Agent Poisoning.

(1) An unexplained runny nose.

(2) Marked difficulty in breathing with tightness in the chest.

(3) Possibly, pinpointed pupils of the eyes.

Note. Upon exposure to vapor or aerosol, the pupils become pinpointed immediately. However, if the nerve agent is only absorbed through the skin or by consuming contaminated food or water, the pinpointing does not occur immediately and may be absent.

(4) Drooling, excessive sweating, nausea, vomiting, cramping, and involuntary urination and defecation.

(5) Jerking, twitching, and staggering.

(6) Headache, confusion, drowsiness, coma, convulsions.

(7) Stoppage of breathing.

Note. If a casualty has the symptoms listed in (4) through (7) above, he probably will not be able to help himself, as they indicate severe poisoning.

c. First Aid Measures for Nerve Agent Poisoning.

(1) Administer atropine. If any of the symptoms of nerve agent poisoning (*b*) above are present, give yourself atropine, using one of your automatic atropine injectors (para 50*b*). This is accomplished as step TWO (para 51*c*(2)). If symptoms persist after 10 to 15 minutes, administer the second injection. If symptoms persist 10 to 15 minutes after the second injection, administer the third injection. If other soldiers are unable to give themselves atropine, inject it for them, using the automatic injectors from their protective mask carriers. Attach each empty injector to the outer clothing to indicate the number of injections received. This can be done by inserting the needle through the clothing and bending it to form a hook.

(*a*) An automatic atropine injector (fig 103) is used as follows:

1. After taking an automatic atropine injector from your protective mask carrier, remove its plastic cover.

Note. By NATO agreement the yellow band circling the self-injection device indicates atropine.

2. Hold the injector in your clenched hand with the yellow safety cap extending above the thumb (a, fig 103).

3. Remove the yellow safety cap by pulling it out (a, fig 103). The automatic injector is now "armed" and ready to use. Do NOT touch the green functioning end until you are ready to give the injection.

4. Place the green end of the injector against the clothing on the outside front thick muscle (thigh) (b, fig 103). Do NOT take time to remove clothing or to expose skin. If you need atropine, *speed is important.*

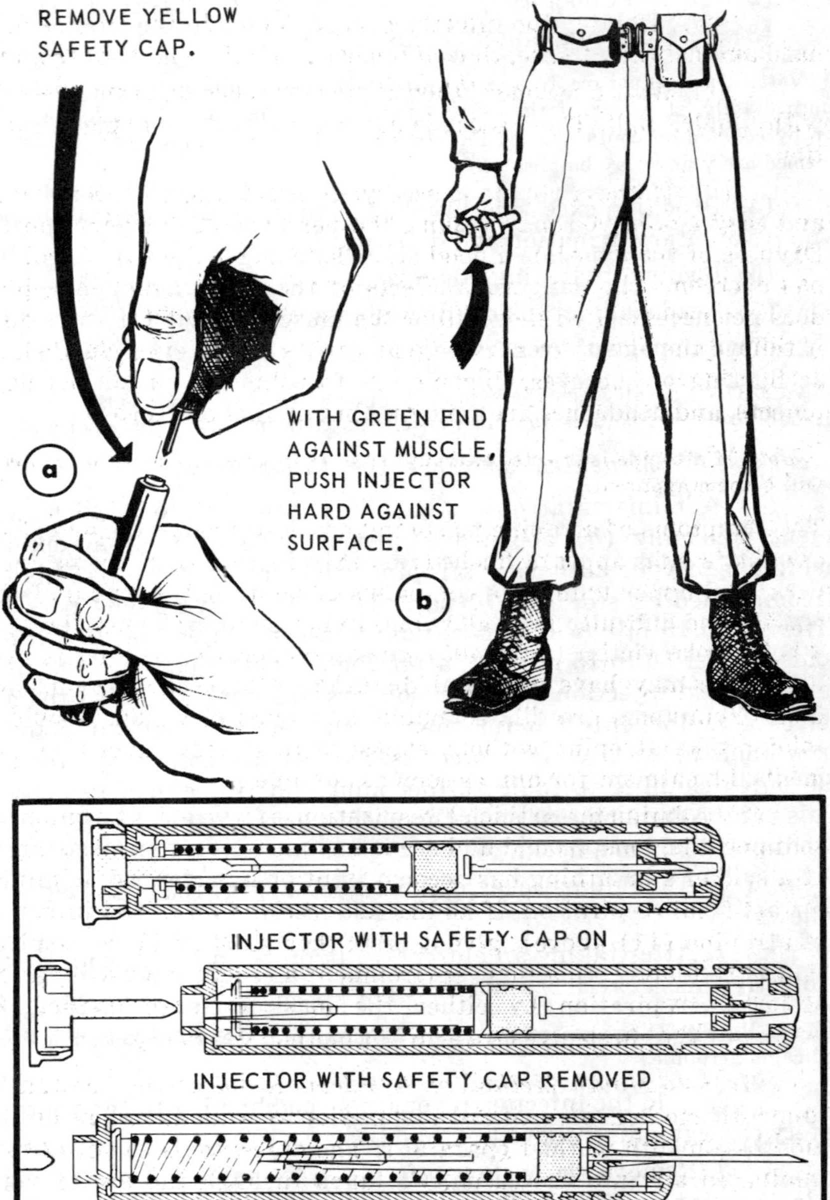

THE PRESSURE EXERTED AUTOMATICALLY ACTIVATES A SPRING WHICH PLUNGES THE INJECTOR NEEDLE INTO THE MUSCLE AND AT THE SAME TIME INJECTS THE 2 MILLIGRAMS OF ATROPINE.

Figure 103. Use of atropine automatic injector.

5. Holding the injector perpendicular to the site, push it hard against the surface, thus automatically injecting the atropine.

6. Wait 5 seconds; then remove the needle from the skin with a quick pull. The 5 seconds are necessary for complete injection.

(*b*) If the atropine causes your breathing to become free and easy again, you may resume the performance of your duties. Dryness of the mouth is a good sign. This means that the atropine has overcome the dangerous effects of the nerve agent. Atropine does not necessarily relieve all of the muscular twitching nor does it relieve the effects of nerve agent vapors in the eyes. Such signs as hurting of the eyes, difficulty in focusing the vision on close objects, and headaches are annoying but are not dangerous.

Note. If atropine is injected without exposure to a nerve agent, toxic effects will become apparent.

The symptoms of atropine poisoning are described as follows: The casualty's skin appears flushed; he may have a rash on his face, neck, and upper trunk. He complains of being hot, dryness of the mouth, and difficulty in swallowing. In hot climates he may become a heatstroke victim (para 40*b*) unless evaporative cooling is provided. He may have a mental disturbance marked by delusions. Other symptoms are dilated pupils and blurred vision. Should a soldier take atropine without exposure to a nerve agent, obtain medical treatment for him as soon as possible.

(2) Administer artificial respiration, if needed. If your mission permits, look around and see if anyone needs your assistance. If a soldier's breathing has become faint or has stopped, administer artificial respiration. If he has not received an initial injection of atropine ((1) above), give it first; then start artificial respiration immediately. In a toxic environment a casualty must be given artificial respiration by either the mask-to-mouth method (*d* below) or the chest-pressure arm-lift method (para 8*c*).

d. Mask-to-Mouth Method of Artificial Respiration. The mask-to-mouth method of artificial respiration is a modification of the mouth-to-mouth method (para 8*b*). The objective is to get uncontaminated air into the casualty's lungs through the use of your M17A1 Field Protective Mask and M1 Resuscitation Tube. The mask-to-mouth method is performed as follows:

(1) Prepare your mask (a, fig 104) for administering artificial respiration:

(*a*) Turn the valve handle (b, fig 104) to the *left,* thus positioning the breathing tube bitepiece (inside the mask) between your teeth.

Note. The breathing tube bitepiece will spring back to the neutral position if you release your bite.

(*b*) Using your left hand, raise the voicemitter cover (a, fig 104); then with your right hand insert the outlet valve of the resuscitation tube (c, fig 104) into the air outlet well which is under the voicemitter cover. To obtain a tight, leakproof seal, first insert the unflanged edge of the air outlet valve (c, fig 104) with an upward push and then press the flanged edge inward as hard as possible.

(*c*) To determine whether or not a leakproof seal has been obtained, fold back and pinch the lower end of the corrugated tube (c, fig 104) and blow into your breathing tube bitepiece. If the corrugated tube does not tend to expand, remove and reinsert the outlet valve as explained in (*b*) above; then check again.

(2) Raise the casualty's protective mask only enough to expose his mouth and nose; then clear his airway (para 7).

(3) Position the casualty on his back, his head in a chin-up position, and his jaw in a jutting-out position as described for mouth-to-mouth (nose) method (para 8*b* (2)–(4)).

(4) Insert and secure the mouthpiece of the resuscitation tube (c, fig 104) between the casualty's lips and teeth (fig 105):

(*a*) To insert the mouthpiece between the casualty's lips and teeth, slide only one-half of it into his mouth at a time. Insert the indented portion of the mouthpiece under the upper lip. Insure that the edges of the mouthpiece are completely sealed with the casualty's lips.

(*b*) Secure the mouthpiece in place by forming a seal over the casualty's lips with your thumb and index finger. Hook the other three fingers under the casualty's chin to keep his jaw in a jutting-out position.

(5) Administer artificial respiration (fig 105):

(*a*) With your free hand, pinch the casualty's nose closed, take a deep breath, and blow into your breathing tube bitepiece ((1)(*a*) above).

(*b*) Continue blowing while watching for the casualty's chest to rise. If his chest does not rise, hold his chin up more forcefully and blow harder. If his chest still does not rise, check all connections for leakage of air.

(*c*) When the casualty's chest rises, stop blowing and release his nose, thus allowing him to exhale. Be sure to close his nose again as soon as he exhales.

(*d*) Continue blowing breaths into the casualty and allowing him to exhale. The first five breaths should be deep and fast to

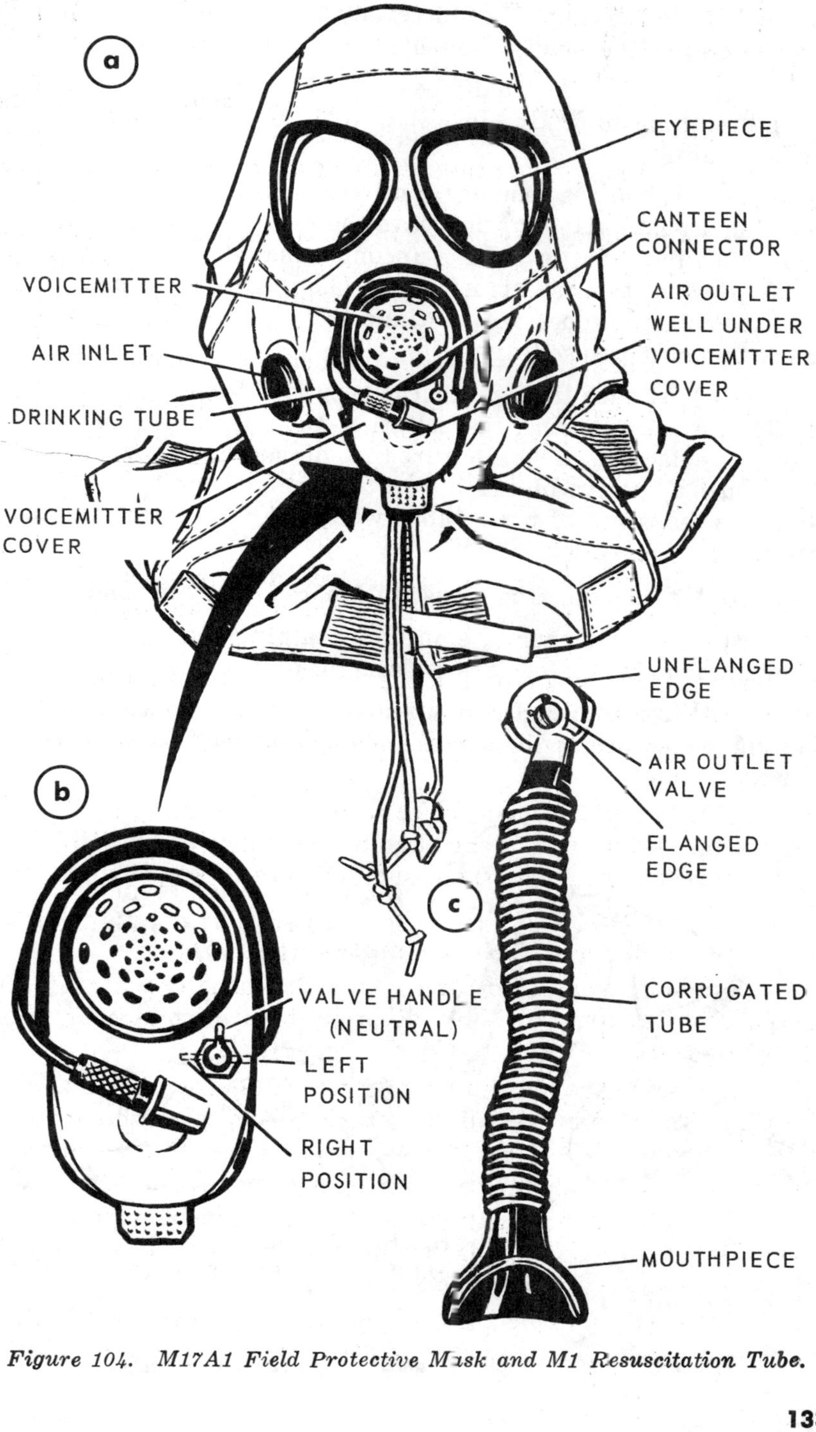

Figure 104. M17A1 Field Protective Mask and M1 Resuscitation Tube.

provide for rapid reoxygenation of blood. Thereafter, the breaths should be blown at a rate of 12 to 20 per minute. If exhalation is noisy, hold the chin up more forcefully or check for the presence of secretions in the casualty's upper airway.

(*e*) When the casualty begins to breathe on his own, adjust your breathing to assist him. Blow when he is inhaling not when he is exhaling.

(*f*) When the casualty continues to breathe regularly, stop blowing air into his lungs but leave the resuscitation tube in place, thus allowing him to inhale uncontaminated air through your mask. Be sure to close his nose when he inhales and open it when he exhales. If he does not continue to breathe regularly, resume mask-to-mouth resuscitation.

(*g*) At such time as the casualty is able to breathe without assistance, remove the resuscitation tube from his mouth and quickly replace his mask. Be sure that his mask is properly sealed. Continue to observe him to insure that he does not stop breathing again as the result of toxic vapor which may have accumulated in his mask.

(6) After completing resuscitation, readjust your mask:

(*a*) Release your bite on the breathing tube bitepiece, thus allowing it to spring back to its *neutral* position (b, fig 104).

(*b*) Disconnect the resuscitation tube from your mask by pulling it outware and upware, and replace the voicemitter cover.

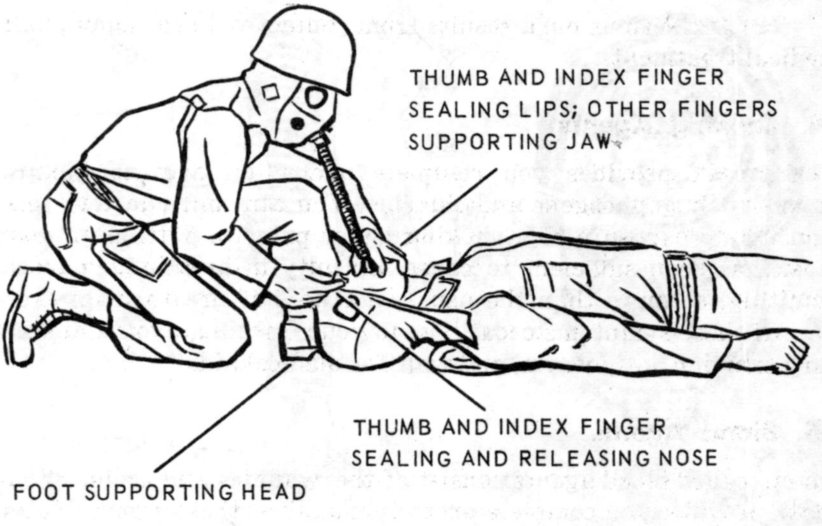

Figure 105. Mask-to-mouth artificial respiration.

(*c*) Wipe the mouthpiece of the resuscitation tube clean and stow it in your carrier.

(7) Notify medical personnel of the casualty's location in accordance with the standing operating procedure of the unit.

53. Blister Agents

a. General. Blister agents (vesicants) include mustards and arsenicals. Relatively low doses may be serious; they can cause serious injury to the eyes, the upper respiratory tract, and the skin. If it is known or suspected that blister agents are being used, you should take cover, mask, and apply powder to your exposed skin, using the skin decontaminating pad from the M13 kit (para 50*c*). If protective clothing has been issued, you should, of course, be wearing it.

b. Symptoms of Blister Agent Poisoning.

(1) *Instant eye pain upon contact with lewisite.* No pain upon contact with mustard.

(2) *Inflammation, blisters, and tissue destruction.* The longer the agent is in contact with the tissue and the larger the area affected, the more serious the injury will become.

c. First Aid Measures for Blister Agent Poisoning. After you have accomplished the applicable steps outlined in paragraph 51*c*, take the following measures as required:

(1) If blisters form, cover them with a loose sterile dressing and secure with bandage (para 16–19) Avoid breaking blisters, if possible.

(2) If a serious burn results from contact with the agent, seek medical treatment.

54. Choking Agents

Your mask provides you complete protection against choking agents such as phosgene and chlorine. You can continue your mission unless exposure to a choking agent prior to putting on your mask has been sufficient to cause difficulty in breathing, nausea, vomiting, or more than the usual shortness of breath upon exertion. If these symptoms occur, loosen your clothing, avoid unnecessary exertion, keep warm, and wait for medical aid.

55. Blood Agents

The so called blood agents consist of the cyanides and arsine. Your mask provides you complete protection against these agents. Exposure to the blood agents before masking, however, can cause rapid, severe interference with your respiration. If exposure to a cyanide blood agent occurs, the first aid measures are inhalation of amyl nitrite and administration of artificial respiration (para 52*d*). Amyl nitrite ampuls may be issued to you in the event that intelligence indicates a blood agent will be used. Rapid action is paramount, since a person's respiration is immediately affected after exposure to such an agent. "Buddy help" will probably be essential. Crush two ampuls of amyl nitrite and place them within the facepiece of the mask. Repeat this procedure at intervals of 4 to 5 minutes, using two ampuls each time, until normal breathing returns or until a total of eight ampuls have been used. *No more should be given,* as amyl nitrite is poisonous and a larger does would be harmful. If a person does not respond to this dose, he needs to be treated further by a medical officer.

56. Tear Agents (CS or CN)

a. Should you be exposed to a tear agent before masking, it can cause an increased flow of tears and intense eye pain; it may irritate the upper respiratory tract. If you mask after exposure, be sure to clear your mask and keep your eyes open as much as possible. When you remove your mask after the all-clear signal, the recovery from the tear agent effects will be spontaneous.

b. If heavy skin contamination occurs in a hot, humid, close environment, blistering may result unless the agent is rinsed from the skin with water. If the agent in liquid or solid form has entered your eyes, force your eyes open and flush them with water. A one-fourth percent solution of sodium sulfite, if available, is more effective in dissolving and neutralizing the irritating agent.

57. Vomiting Agents

DM (Adamsite), DA, and DC typify this group of agents. Your mask provides you protection against them. Exposure to such an agent before masking may cause sneezing, nausea, salivation, and vomiting but are not dangerous to healthy individuals. If excessive salivation or vomiting makes lifting your mask necessary, be sure to clear your mask after you reseat it. Vigorous activity help reduce nausea and its duration.

58. Incapacitating Agents

Generally speaking, an incapacitating agent is any compound which can interfere with the performance of military duties by affecting the central nervous system and by producing muscular weakness and abnormal behavior. It is likely that such agents will be disseminated by smoke-producing munitions or aerosols, thus making breathing their means of entry into the body. The use of the protective mask is, therefore, essential for protection against the agents.

a. There is no special first aid for the relief of the symptoms of incapacitating agents. Supportive first aid and physical restraint may be indicated. Weapons and other potentially harmful materials should be removed from the possession of individuals who are suspected casualties. This includes cigarettes, matches, medications, and small items which might be swallowed accidentally. Delirious patients have been known to attempt to eat items bearing only a superficial resemblance to food.

b. Anticholinergic poisoning (BZ type) may produce alarming dryness and coating of the lips and tongue; however there is usually no danger of immediate dehydration. Fluids should be given sparingly, if at all, because of the danger of vomiting and because of the likelihood of temporary urinary retention due to paralysis of bladder muscles. An important medical consideration is the possibility of heatstroke because of stoppage of sweating (para 40*b*). If the environmental temperature is above 78°F., remove excessive clothing from the casualty and dampen him to allow evaporative cooling and prevent dehydration. If the casualty does not readily improve, apply first aid measure for heatstroke (para 40*b*) and seek medical attention.

59. Screening Smokes

a. *Titanium Tetrachloride* (*FM*) *Smoke*. This smoke is relatively nontoxic, but the liquid burns the skin like a strong acid. The smoke is irritating to the nose and throat but only mildly so at the concentration usually found in a smoke cloud. The protective mask should be worn in heavy concentrations of FM. Flush any liquid FM from the skin with water.

b. *Sulfur Trioxide-Chlorosulfonic Acid Solution* (*FS*) *Smoke*. Smoke of this solution causes a prickling sensation on the skin because of the minute acid particles of which it is composed. Liquid FS is highly corrosive to the skin. Splashes of liquid FS in the eyes produces extremely painful acid burns. Exposure to heavy concentrations or prolonged exposure to ordinary concentrations may cause severe irritation of the eyes, the skin, and the respiratory tract. The protective mask should be worn in high FS smoke concentrations. Flush any liquid FS from the skin and eyes with water from your canteen (para 51*c*(3)).

c. HC Mixture (HC). This smoke in high concentrations such as might be encountered near an operating munition, in an inclosed space, or near dense HC smoke screens and in ordinary field concentrations for a prolonged period may have a sufficient amount of zinc chloride built up to produce toxic effects. The protective mask should, therefore, be worn. The effects of exposure to HC may include irritation of the nose and throat, coughing, choking, headache, fever, chest and muscular pains, and suffocation. If nausea, vomiting, or difficulty in breathing occurs, get medical aid as soon as conditions permit. Aspirin will ease general discomfort.

d. Oil Smoke. Inhalation of oil smoke produces no apparent symptoms immediately even though it is inhaled for extended periods. Operating personnel exposed to prolonged high concentrations of oil smoke should wear protective masks as much of the time as possible.

e. White Phosphorus (WP) Smoke. This smoke is harmless; however injuries from burning solid or liquid WP are serious. These burns heal very slowly. For first aid measures, see paragraph 60*a*.

60. Incendiaries

Incendiaries can be grouped as white phosphorous, thickened fuel, metal, and oil and metal. You must learn to protect yourself against these types of incendiaries.

a. White phosphorus (WP) is used primarily as a smoke producer but can be used for its incendiary effect to ignite field expedients and combustible flame material. The burns from WP are usually multiple, deep, and variable in size. When particles of WP get on the skin or clothing, they continue to burn until deprived of air. They also have a tendency to stick to a surface and must be brushed off or picked out. Should burning WP strike you—

(1) Smother the flame by submerging yourself in water or by dousing the WP with water from your canteen or any other source. Urine, a wet cloth, or mud can be used. Copper sulfate pads, if available, can be wet and put over the burning WP. The copper sulfate reacts chemically to coat the phosphorus particles and to prevent further activity. You may be able to take off contaminated clothing quickly before the phosphorus burns through to the skin.

Note. Since WP is poisonous to the system, grease or oil should NOT be used to smother the flame because the WP will be absorbed into the body with the grease or oil.

(2) Keep the WP particles covered with wet material to ex-

clude air until you can remove them or get them removed from your skin.

(3) Remove the WP particles from the skin by brushing them with a wet cloth and by picking them out with a knife, bayonet, stick, or similar object.

(4) Report to a medical facility for treatment as soon as your mission permits.

b. Thickened fuel mixtures (napalm) have a tendency to cling to the clothing and the body surfaces, thereby producing prolonged exposures and severe burns. The first aid for these burns is the same as for other heat burns (para 25 and 34). The heat and irritating gases given off by these combustible mixtures may cause lung damage which must be treated by a medical officer.

c. Metal incendiaries pose special problems. Thermite and thermate particles on the skin should be immediately cooled with water from your canteen and then removed. Even though thermate particles have their own oxygen supply and continue to burn under water, it helps to cool them with water. The first aid for these burns is the same as for other heat burns (para 25). Particles of magnesium on the skin burn quickly and deeply. Like the other metal incendiaries, they must be removed. Ordinarily, the complete removal of these particles should be done by trained personnel at a medical treatment facility, using local anesthesia. The casualty needs medical treatment immediately.

d. Oil and metal incendiaries have much the same effect on contact with the skin and clothing as those discussed in *b* and *c* above. Appropriate first aid measures are described in paragraph 25.

CHAPTER 7
PSYCHOLOGICAL FIRST AID

61. General

a. Importance of Psychological First Aid. You have learned that first aid is the emergency measures which you can apply before trained medical personnel arrive. First aid can be applied to injuries of the mind as well as to those of the body. You must, therefore, know how to give psychological first aid in order to help yourself, your buddies, and your unit to keep fighting. An emotional upset which results in poor judgment can be just as fatal as a bullet in the heart. It can be even more dangerous if other persons are affected by the judgment of an emotionally upset person.

b. Explanation of the Term "Psychological First Aid." Psychological first aid is as natural and reasonable as physical first aid and is as familiar if you stop to think about it. When you were hurt as a child, the understanding attitude of your parents did as much as the "Band Aid" or the "Mercurochrome" to ease the pain. Later on, disappointment or grief was eased by encouraging words from a friend. Certainly, taking a walk and talking things out with a friend are familiar ways of dealing with an emotional crisis. The same natural feelings that make us want to help a person who is injured make us want to give a helping hand to a buddy who is feeling emotionally "all shook up." You see, psychological first aid really means nothing more complicated than helping people with emotional injuries whether they result from physical injury, disease, or excessive or unbearable strain on their emotions. Emotional injuries are not as visible as a wound, a broken leg, or a reaction to pain from physical damage; but severe fear, excessive worry, depression, or overexcitement is evidence that emotional damage has occurred. The more noticeable the symptom, the more urgent the need is for you to be of help and the more important it is for you to know how to help.

c. Situations in Which Psychological First Aid May Be Needed. The situations which present the greatest need for psychological first aid are those in which trained medical personnel are not immediately available. These situations occur in combat and civilian disasters such as floods, hurricanes, and catastrophes of nuclear warfare. Although it is worthwhile to remember that emotional reactions are temporary, lasting only for minutes, hours, or at the most a few days, they are seriously disabling, are often contagious, and may result in danger not only to the emotionally upset individual but also to the entire unit. In such situations you may be working alongside of someone who cannot handle the impact of disaster upon his emotions. Even when there is no danger of physical injury, psychological injury may occur.

d. Interrelation of Psychological First Aid and Physical First Aid. Psychological first aid often goes hand in hand with physical first aid. The discovery of a physical injury does not rule out the possibility of a psychological injury. A physical injury and the circumstances surrounding it may actually cause an emotional injury. Both need treatment. The person suffering from pain, shock, fears of serious damage to his body, or even death does not respond well to joking, indifference, or fearful-tearful attention. Fear and anxiety may take as high a toll of the casualty's strength as does the loss of blood.

e. Goals of Psychological First Aid. Simply stated, the goals of psychological first aid are to—

(1) Return the casualty to duty in as short a period as possible.

(2) Minimize his immediate disability even though prompt return to duty is not possible.

(3) Decrease the intensity of his emotional reaction until more complete care, if needed, can be arranged.

(4) Prevent actions harmful to him and to the efforts of others.

62. Four Principles To Remember

Just as no one expects you to substitute for a surgeon, it is not planned that you replace medical personnel in this area either; but your help can be of great value until more qualified personnel become available. Effective first aid will help get the psychological casualty back into action sooner. An emotional reaction should not be too strange to you because you probably have had some inkling of an emotional reaction yourself or have seen something like it before—although perhaps not so severe. Here are a few principles that will make your first aid job easier.

a. Respect Everyone's Right To Have His Own Feelings.

(1) Accept the casualty whom you are trying to help without

censorship or ridicule. Accept his right to his own feelings. Just because your feelings, beliefs, and behavior are different, do not blame or make light of him for the way he feels or acts. Your job is to help him in this tough situation, not to be his critic. A person does not want to be upset and worried; he would "snap out of it" if he could. When he seeks help, he needs and expects consideration of his fears, not abrupt dismissal, chidings, or accusations. You may be impressed with the fact that you made it through in good conditions, but you have no guarantee that the situation will not be reversed next time.

(2) Realize that people are the products of a wide variety of factors. All persons do not react the same way to the same situation. Each individual has complex needs and motivations, both conscious and unconscious, that are uniquely his own; thus an injury or an emotional catastrophe will have a personal meaning for each. Even though you may not share the reactions or feelings of another person and even though the reactions seem foolish or peculiar, you must realize that he feels this way for a reason. You can help him most by accepting this fact and by doing what you can for him during this difficult time. He is doing the best he can under the circumstances. You must help him the best you can.

b. Accept Emotional Disability As Being Just As Real As Physical Disability.

(1) If a soldier's leg is blown off by a landmine, no one (including the wounded man himself) expects him to walk right away. If a soldier's emotions are shattered by the overwhelming stress of more "blood and guts" than he can take for a while or by the explosion of a nuclear bomb, many people seem inclined to expect him to pull himself together immediately and carry on without a break. Some individuals can do this, but some cannot. Those who cannot have just as real a disability as the soldier who has lost his leg. There is an unfortunate tendency in many people to regard as real only those things they can see, such as wound, bleeding, or an X-ray picture of a diseased lung. Most people tend to assume that damage which involves the mind and emotions is probably just imagined, that the person is not really sick or injured, and that he could overcome his trouble by using his willpower.

(2) The terms, "It's all in your head," "Snap out of it," "Buck up," and "Get control of yourself" are often used by people who believe they are being helpful. Actually, these terms are expressions of hostility because they show lack of understanding. They only "goad" and emphasize weakness and inadequacy. Such terms are of no use in psychological first aid. A psychological casualty or a physical casualty with strong emotional reactions to his injury

does not want to feel as he does. He would like to be effective, but he is temporarily overcome with fear and anxiety. He feels lost and unable to control his emotions for awhile. Reminding him of his failure to act as others do only "rubs salt into the wound."

c. Realize That Every Physically Injured Person Has Some Emotional Reaction to the Fact That He Is Injured.

(1) A slight injury such as a cut finger gives most people a start. It is normal for an injured person to feel upset. The more severe the injury, the more insecure and fearful he becomes, especially if the injury is to a body part which is highly valued. For example, an injury to the eyes or the genitals, even though a relatively minor one, is likely to be severely upsetting. An injury to some other part of the body may be especially disturbing to an individual for his own particular reason. For example, an injury of the hand may be a terrifying blow to a baseball pitcher or a pianist; a facial disfigurement may be especially threatening to an actor.

(2) An injured person always feels less secure, more anxious, and more afraid not only because of what has happened to him but also because of more dire things he imagines may still happen as a result of his injury. This fear and insecurity may cause him to be irritable, stubborn, or unreasonable he may seem uncooperative, unnecessarily difficult, or even emotionally irrational. As you help him, always keep in mind that such behavior has little or nothing to do with you personally. He needs your patience, reassurance, encouragement, and support. Even though he seems disagreeable and ungrateful at first, get across the idea that you want to help him.

d. Realize There Is More Strength in Most Disturbed Soldiers Than Appears at First Glance. No injured or sick person puts his best foot forward. The strong points of his personality are likely to be hidden beneath his fear, anguish, and pain. It is easy to see only his failures even though he worked efficiently alongside of you only a short time ago. With your aid he will be helping you or someone else again. Whatever made him a good soldier, rifleman, or buddy is still there. He is needed.

63. Common Types of Reactions to Disaster

a. Normal. Most people react to a disaster (military or civilian, personal or public, threatened or actual) by doing something about it immediately or within a few minutes after they "collect" themselves. With a few exceptions all people feel some fear. This fear may be greater than that experienced at any other time, or they may be more aware of their fear. In such a situation you should not be surprised if you feel shaky, perspire profusely, and become a little nauseated and confused. These reactions are normal and are not cause for concern. After a while, if you get busy, your heart will stop pounding, your breath will come back, and you will feel less tense.

b. Abnormal Reactions. Some reactions can be easily recognized as abnormal. The following are the most usual:

(1) *Physical reactions.* Some of the reactions to a disaster can be seen or felt physically in the form of bodily changes such as rapid breathing, fast pulse, "butterflies" in the stomach, and shakiness. Some or all of these may appear before the disaster actually happens, or they may not appear until the disaster occurs. If any of these symptoms become severe, they may prevent effective performance of duty. A severely nauseated soldier cannot man a machine gun; a person who is convinced that he cannot see is not able to drive a truck; a soldier who believes his leg is paralyzed is a burden to his buddies.

(2) *Panic reactions.* You can easily understand that overwhelming fear can cause some people to act in abnormal ways. You can remember how you felt or how others acted when severely frightened. Some seem to lose all control and do things in a blind, unreasonable way. They may run aimlessly with complete disregard for their safety, may weep so severely they become exhausted and unable to care for themselves even when their lives depend upon it, or may recklessly go about doing things that make no sense.

(3) *Overactive reactions.* In disaster situations you can expect "running about" and confusion. Some people, however, seem to run about, creating additional confusion and doing things that are of no value or even harmful. They talk a lot, make silly jokes, or may be demanding, critical, and overly confident. You can see them jump from job to job, brush aside any directions, and make a spectacle of themselves.

(4) *Depressed reactions.* Most people are dazed, shocked, or numb after a disaster but this condition promptly clears up. Sometimes, however, a person will not be able "to shake it off." He acts as if he were alone in the world. When he moves, if he does, his movements are slow and aimless. He will hardly respond to anyone or anything and will show no emotion at all—only a vacant stare. A person like this is completely helpless and unaware of his surroundings.

c. Helpful Hints in Recognizing Emotional Reactions. You do not need much training to recognize severe abnormal reactions. There are other soldiers, however, who will have reactions that are less severe and more difficult to detect. To determine whether or not a man needs help, find out if he is doing something which makes sense and if he is able to perform his duties and take care of himself. You probably will make it through all right, but it will help you to stop for a moment and check yourself. You may need to slow down or to get going.

64. First Aid Measures

Psychological first aid measures are simple and easy to understand. Improvisation is in order, just as it is in splinting a fracture. Your judgment as to what to do depends upon your ability to observe the casualty and understand the needs to be met. Time is on your side and so are the resources of the soldier whom you are helping. How to make the best use of his resources is your problem.

a. Getting Through. The emotionally disturbed casualty has erected a barrier against fear. If he finds that he does not have to be afraid and that there are normal, understandable things about him, he will feel safer in dropping this barrier. Persistent efforts to make him realize that you want to understand him will be reassuring. Familiar things such as a cup of coffee, the use of his name, attention to even a minor wound, or the sight of familiar people and activities will add to his ability to overcome his fear. He will not respond well if you are excited, angry, or abrupt.

b. Ventilation. Everyone needs to communicate with others. There is no better medicine for fear and feelings of isolation than a chance to talk with a friendly person. Encourage talk and be a good listener. Find out what happened to him. Let him answer in his own way. It is neither possible nor desirable for you to allow endless rambling; but his feelings of helplessness and despair will often be relieved remarkably if you will give him a few minutes to talk about his own experiences and fears. Give him time to tell what happened to him, what he thinks happened to him, or what he fears may still happen to him. A person will frequently solve his own problem when he is encouraged to put it into his own words and to examine how he really feels about it. In the terror of injury, of battle, or of catastrophe, many casualties give up. By being calm, patient, and willing to listen, you can get across the idea that you believe in him, that you respect him as a human being, and that you think he is worthwhile. If he understands that help is available, beginning with you, it will do wonders to reestablish his faith in himself and to help him "to get his feet on solid ground." Most emotional casualties, even severely disturbed ones, make remarkable recoveries when they are helped to face themselves and to reorganize their shattered feelings. They become able to turn their attention from themselves to others.

c. Activity.

(1) A person who is emotionally disturbed due to combat or catastrophe is basically a casualty of fear. He is disabled because he has become temporarily overwhelmed by fear. The best way to get rid of fear is through action: doing something about the situation; moving against the force or thing that threatens; being active, aggressive, or helpful and consequently feeling needed, useful, and successful. Almost all soldiers, for example, experience a considerable sense of fear while they are poised, awaiting the opening of a big offensive; but this is normally relieved and they actually feel better once they begin to move into action. They take pride in effective performance and pleasure in knowing that they are good soldiers, perhaps being completely unaware that overcoming their fears was their first accomplishment.

(2) This same measure can be applied very effectively to many psychological casualties who are not physically incapacitated. After you help a casualty to get over his initial fear, to regain some self-confidence, and to realize his job is to continue to function as best he can, you should then help him find something useful to do. Encourage him to be active. Get him to carry litters, help load trucks, clean up debris, dig fox holes, or assist with refugees. If possible, get him back to his usual duty. Seek out his strong points and help him to apply them. Avoid having him just sit around. You will have to provide direction by telling him what to do and where to do it. The instructions should be clear and simple; they should be repeated; they should be reasonable and obviously possible. A person who is in panic is likely to argue. Respect his feelings but point out more immediate, obtainable, and demanding needs. Channel his excessive energy, and above all do not argue. If you cannot get him interested in doing more profitable work, it may be necessary to enlist aid in controlling his overactivity before it spreads to the group and results in more panic. Prevent the spread of such infectious feelings by restraining and segregating if necessary.

(3) Involvement in activity helps a casualty in three ways: He forgets himself; he has an outlet for his excessive tensions; and he proves to himself he can do something useful. It is amazing how effective this is in helping a person to overcome feelings of fear, ineffectiveness, and uselessness.

d. Rest. There are times, particularly in combat, when physical exhaustion is a principal cause for emotional reactions. For the weary, dirty soldier, adequate rest, warm food, and a change of clothes with an opportunity to bathe may provide spectacular results.

e. Usefulness of Group Spirit. You have probably already noticed that a person works better, faces danger better, and handles serious problems better in a group. Each individual in a group supports the others and seems to be strengthened in turn by the group. For example, you can see the group spirit in the football team and in the school fraternity as well as in the gang that is up to some devilment. Because the individuals share the same interest, goals, and problems, they do more and better work; furthermore they are less worried because everyone is helping. It is this group spirit that wins games, elects majors, and takes a strategic hill in battle. It is so powerful that it is one of the most effective tools you have in psychological first aid. Getting the soldier back into the group and letting him see its orderly and effective activity will reestablish his sense of belonging and security and will go far toward making him a useful member of the unit again.

65. Your Reactions and Limitations

a. Up to this point the discussion has been primarily about the feelings of the psychological casualty. What about your feelings toward him? Whatever the situation, you will have emotional reactions (consciously or unconsciously) toward this casualty. Your reactions can either help or hinder your ability to help him. Especially when you are tired or worried, you may very easily become impatient with the person who seems to be "dragging his heels" or "making mountains out of molehills." You may even feel resentful toward him. At times when many wounded lie about you, it will be especially natural for you to resent disabilities that you cannot see. Physical wounds can be seen and easily accepted. Emotional reactions are more difficult to accept as injuries. On the other hand, will you tend to be overly sympathetic? Excessive sympathy for an incapacitated person can be as harmful as negative feelings in your relationship with him. He needs strong help but not your sorrow. To overwhelm him with pity will make him feel even more inadequate. You must expect your buddy to recover, to be able to return to duty, and to become a useful soldier. This expectation should be displayed in your behavior and attitude as well as in what you say. If he can see in you calmness, confidence, and competence, he will be reassured and will feel greater security in the world around him.

b. Above all, you must guard against becoming impatient, intolerant, and resentful on one hand and overly solicitous on the other. Remember that such emotion in you will rarely help the casualty and can never increase your ability to make clear decisions. A physically injured person can sometimes continue to help others; but an emotionally injured one cannot help others.

c. The same as with the physically injured casualty, the medical personnel will take over the care of the psychological casualty as soon as possible. The first aid which he has received from you will be of great value to his recovery.

66. Summary

a. Learn to detect abnormal reactions in an individual who has undergone stressful situations and keep aware of the importance of psychological first aid to his recovery. Remember that your help can be of great value.

b. Realize that a casualty with an emotional disability is just as truly sick as a physically disabled one and just as able to recover if he is given the proper care.

c. Accept the casualty's reactions and feelings as the best he can do under the circumstances. Realize that he cannot change without help; otherwise he would.

d. Find effective ways of making contact with the casualty. In doing so, take into consideration the facts that he is disturbed, excessively frightened, and overly worried and that he has lost his ability to act as other persons do. By your words, attitude, and behavior, let him know of your willingness and ability to understand his feelings. Show patience and real desire to help.

e. Help him to regain his confidence and to feel more secure in the world about him. Assure him that you expect him to recover fully, that there is much he can do, and that there is a pressing need for his help.

APPENDIX A

REFERENCES

AR 310–5	Dictionary of United States Army Terms.
AR 310–50	Authorized Abbreviations and Brevity Codes.
FM 21–10	Military Sanitation.
FM 21–40	Chemical, Biological, Radiological and Nuclear Defense.
FM 21–41	Soldier's Handbook for Defense Against Chemical and Biological Operations and Nuclear Warfare.

APPENDIX B

CONTENTS OF FIRST AID CASE, KITS, AND PACKS

1. First Aid Case (Individual)

Nomenclature	*Unit*	*Quantity*
Dressing, First Aid, Field, 4 x 7 inches	ea	1
Sodium Chloride-Sodium Bicarbonate Mixture	pg	2

2. General Purpose First Aid Kit

(Available in Vehicles)

Nomenclature	*Unit*	*Quantity*
Ammonia Inhalant Solution, Aromatic, Ampuls, ⅓ cc., 10s	pg	1
Benzalkonium Chloride, Tincture, Tinted, 1:1000, 2cc.	bt	4
Bandage, Absorbent Adhesive, ¾ by 3 inches, 18s	pg	1
Compress, Gauze, 2 by 2 inches, 4s	pg	1
Compress, Gauze, 4 by 4 inches	ea	1
First Aid Kit, Eye Dressing	ea	1
Bandage, Gauze, Compressed, 4 inches by 6 yards	ea	1
Bandage, Muslin, Compressed, 37 by 37 by 52 inches	ea	1
Pin, Safety, Curved, Orthopedic, Medium, 12s	pg	1
Instruction Card, Artificial Respiration, Mouth-to-Mouth Resuscitation	ea	1
Instruction Sheet, First Aid	ea	1

3. Airplane First Aid Kit

(Available in Aircraft)

Nomenclature	*Unit*	*Quantity*
Benzalkonium Chloride Tincture, Tinted, 1:1000, 2 cc.	bt	2
Bandage, Absorbent, Adhesive, ¾ by 3 inches, 18s	pg	1
Dressing, First Aid, Field, 4 by 7 inches	ea	1
Dressing, First Aid, Field, 7½ by 8 inches	ea	2
Compress, Gauze, 4 by 4 inches	ea	1
Gauze, Petrolatum, 3 by 36 inches, 3s	pg	1
First Aid Kit, Eye Dressing	ea	1
Tourniquet, Nonpneumatic, 1½ by 42 inches	ea	1
Blade, Surgical Preparation Razor, Straight, Single Edge, 5s	pg	1
Water Purification Tablet, Iodine, 8 mg., 50s	bt	1

4. Emergency Medical Treatment Unit—Phase I

This unit is comprised of seven subunits or packs as follows: four identical wound packs, two identical burn packs, and one fracture pack. The content of each type of pack is given below and is subject to change at any time.

a. Wound Pack.

Nomenclature	*Unit*	*Quantity*
Dressing, First-Aid, Field, 4 by 7 inches	ea	48
Compress and Bandage, Field, 18 by 22-inch Compress	ea	8
Sponge, Surgical, 4 by 4 inches, 200s	pg	3
Bandage, Gauze, Roller, 4 inches by 10 yards, 12s	pg	3
Scissors, Bandage, Angular, Lister, 7¼-inch	ea	1
Pin, Safety, Curved, Orthopedic, Large, 12s	pg	3
*Airway, Pharyngeal, Plastic, Adult-Child	ea	1

b. Burn Packs.

Nomenclature	*Unit*	*Quantity*
Gauze, Absorbent, 36 inches by 5 yards	pg	18
Bandage, Gauze, Roller, 4 inches by 10 yards, 12s	pg	2
Scissors, Bandage, Angular, Lister, 7¼-inch	ea	1
Pin, Safety, Curved, Orthopedic, Large, 12s	pg	6
Sodium Chloride-Sodium Bicarbonate Mixture, 4.5 Gm., 2s	pg	96
Lubricant, Surgical, 4 oz. (113.4 Gm.)	tu	60
*Airway, Pharyngeal, Plastic, Adult-Child	ea	1

c. Fracture Pack.

Nomenclature	*Unit*	*Quantity*
Wadding, Cotton, Surgical, Sheet, 5 inches by 6 yards, 12s	pg	6
Bandage, Muslin, Compressed, 37 by 37 by 52 inches	ea	5
Bandage, Gauze, Roller, 4 inches by 10 yards, 12s	pg	4
Scissors, Bandage, Angular, Lister, 7¼-inch	ea	1
Splint, Wire, Ladder, 3½ by 31 inches	ea	36
Pin, Safety, Curved, Orthopedic, Large, 12s	pg	3
*Airways, Pharyngeal, Plastic, Adult-Child	ea	1

*These items are to be used only by persons who have had special training in how to use them.

INDEX

	Paragraph	Page
Airway:		
Clearing of	7	10
Defined	4*b*(1)	6
Amyl nitrate ampuls	55	135
Arteries	4*a*(2)(*a*)	4
Artificial respiration, methods of:		
Chest-pressure arm-lift	8*c*, 52*e*(2)	16, 131
Mask-to-mouth	8*b*, 52*d*	11, 131
Mouth-to-mouth	8*b*	11
Mouth-to-nose	8*b*	11
Atropine injector, automatic	50*b*, 51*c*(2)–(6), 52*c*	126, 127, 129
Bandages:		
Cravat	18*b*	36
Roller	18*c*	37
Tailed	18*a*	36
Triangular	18*b*	36
Bandaging of body parts:		
Abdomen	24*b*(1)	70
Back	19*e*	51
Chest	19*e*, 23*b*(2)(*b*)	51, 69
Ear	19*b*	43
Elbow	19*g*	53
Eyes	19*b*	43
Fingers	19*j*	61
Foot	19*m*	64
Forearm	19*h*	55
Hand	19*i*	57
Head	19*a*	39
Hip	19*f*	53
Jaw	19*c*	46
Knee	19*k*	62
Leg	19*l*	62
Shoulder	19*d*	49
Biological agents, protection from	50–51	125
Bleeding, stoppage of	5*b*, 10–12, 14*b*	6, 24, 31
Blood:		
Circulation	4*a*	4
Flow	4*a*(2)(*a*)–(*c*)	4
Vessels	4*a*(2)	4

	Paragraph	Page
Burns:		
Incendiaries, from	60	138
Minor	34	92
Screening smokes, from	59	137
Severe	25	71
Canteen cover, M1 protective	25*b*(2)(*c*)	73
Capillaries	4*a*(2)(*c*)	5
Carbon:		
Dioxide	4*b*	5
Monoxide poisoning	42	100
Carrying of casualty, methods for:		
Arms carry	48*d*	110
Back lift and carry	48*g*	113
Fireman's carry	48*b*	109
Four-hand:		
Arms carry	48*o*	120
Packsaddle carry	48*m*	120
Neck drag	48*j*	117
Pack-strap carry	48*f*	112
Pistol-belt:		
Carry	48*h*	115
Drag	48*i*	115
Saddleback carry	48*e*	111
Supporting carry	48*c*	110
Two-man:		
Arms carry	48*l*	119
Saddleback carry	48*m*	120
Supporting carry	48*k*	119
Chemical agents:		
Blister	53	135
Blood	55	135
Choking	54	135
Incapacitating	58	136
Incendiaries	60	138
Nerve	52	128
Screening smokes	59	137
Tear	56	136
Vomiting	57	136
Chemical attack, first aid steps for	51*c*	127
Chest cage	4*b*(3), 9*b*	6, 18
Closed-chest heart massage	8*a*(2), 9	10, 18
Constrictive clothing, loosening of	14*c*, 40*a*(1)	31, 97
Digital pressure	11*c*(2)	27
Disaster:		
Reactions to	63, 65	143, 147
Supplies for	6*d*	7
Dislocations	27*a*	73
Dressing of wounds	11, 16–17, 21*b*(1), 23*b*(2)(*a*), 24*b*(1), 25*b*(1)(*b*), 33	24, 33, 67, 68, 70, 72, 92

	Paragraph	Page
Drowning	43	100
Ear, foreign body in	36*a*	94
Electric shock	44	101
Elevation of injured part	11*c*(1)	24
Emergency medical treatment unit (*See* First aid, unit.)		
Emotional injuries	61	140
Equipment (*See* First aid, equipment.)		
Exhalation	4*b*	5
Eye, foreign body in	35	93
First aid:		
Case, individual	6*a*, app B	7, 150
Equipment for toxic environment	50	125
Importance of	3, 6*d*, 49*b*, 61*a*	3, 7, 140
Kit:		
Airplane	6*c*, app B	7, 150
General purpose	6*b*, app B	7, 150
M13	50*c*	126
Measures:		
Common emergency	33–45	92
Lifesaving	7–19	10
Psychological	61–66	140
Special	20–32	67
Toxic environment	51*c*–60	126
Unit for emergency medical treatment, phase I	6*d*, app B	7, 150
Foot:		
Immersion	41*b*	98
Trouble	37	94
Fractures:		
Closed	27*a*	73
Open	27*b*	73
Signs of	28–29	73
Splinting and immobilizing:		
Bandages for	31*c*	78
Collarbone	32*c*(2)	80
Importance of	29	75
Improvisation of	31*a*	77
Jaw	32*c*(1)	79
Lower extremities	32*b*	79
Neck	32*e*	87
Padding for	31*b*	78
Ribs	32*c*(4)	81
Rules for	30	75
Shoulder	32*c*(3)	81
Slings for	31*d*	78
Spinal column	32*d*	83
Upper extremities	32*c*	78
Wire ladder for	31*c*	77
Frostbite	41*c*	99

	Paragraph	Page
Heart:		
Defined	4*a*(1)	4
Massage, closed chest	9	18
Heat:		
Cramps	40*c*	98
Exhaustion	40*a*	97
Heatstroke	40*b*, 52*c*(1)(*b*), 58*b*	97, 131, 137
Immersion foot	41*b*	98
Infection, prevention of	5*d*, 15, 25*b*(1), 29, 33, 34*a*, 37, 41*c*(2)(*b*)	7, 33, 71, 75, 92, 94, 99
Inhalation	4*b*	5
Kit (*See* First aid, kit.)		
Life-saving measures:		
A	5*a*, 7–9	6, 10
B	5*b*, 10–12	6, 24
C	5*c*, 13–14	6, 31
D	5*d*, 15–19	7, 33
Litters, improvised	47	106
Lungs	4*b*(2)	6
Maintenance of manual	2	3
Markings for casualty	12*e*	30
Mask, field protective	25*b*(2)(*c*), 50*a*, 51*a*, 52*d*, 55, 57, 59	73, 126, 131, 135, 136, 137
Masking, conditions for	51	126
Measures, first aid (*See* First aid, measures.)		
Nose, foreign body in	36*b*	94
One-man carry	48*b*–*j*	109
Oxygen	4*b*, 5*a*	5, 6
Pain, relief of	14*h*	33
Poisoning:		
Carbon monoxide	42	100
Chemical agents	49–60	125
Plants, from	39	97
Poisoning of casualty with/for:		
Abdominal wound	24*b*(3)	70
Artificial respiration	8*b*–*c*	11
Chest, sucking wound of	23*b*(3)	69
Closed-chest heart massage	9*c*	19
Face wound	22*b*(2)	68
Fractures	30*a*, 32*d*–*e*	75, 83
Head injury	21*b*(3)	68

	Paragraph	Page
Neck wound	22*b*(2)	68
Shock control	14*f*	32
Snake bite	38*a*(2)	96
Pressure points	11*c*(2)	27
Prickly heat	40	97
Psychological first aid:		
Defined	61*b*	140
Goals of	61*e*	141
Importance of	61*a*	140
Measures	64	145
Needs for	61*c*–*d*	140
Principles of	62	141
Reactions requiring	63*b*–*c*	144
Pulse	4*a*(2)(*a*), 9*a*	4, 18
Purpose of manual	1	3
Rate of:		
Artificial respiration	8*b*(6)(*d*), 8*c*(5)(*c*)	14
Closed-chest heart massage	9*c*(3)(*c*)	20
Pulse	4*a*(2)(*a*)	4
Respiration	4*b*(3)	6
Reassuring casualty	14*d*	31
References	app A	149
Respiration:		
Artificial	8, 52*d*	10, 131
Defined	4*b*	5
Scorpion sting	38*c*	96
Shock:		
Control	13–14, 25*b*(2), 28	31, 72, 73
Defined	5*c*	6
Electric	44	101
Skin eruption from plants	39	97
Snake bite	38*a*	95
Snow blindness	41*d*	99
Sodium chloride—sodium bicarbonate	25*b*(2), app B	72, 150
Spider bite	38*b*	96
Splinting of fracture (*See* Fracture, splinting.)		
Sprains	27*a*	73
Sunburn	34, 40	92, 97
Sunstroke (*See* Heatstroke.)		
Supplies (*See* First aid.)		
Throat, foreign body in	36*c*	94
Tourniquet:		
Application of	12, 38*a*(3)	27, 96
Inspection of	12*f*	30

	Paragraph	Page
Toxic environment:		
Protection from	50–51	125
First aid for:		
Blister agents	53*c*	135
Blood agents	55	135
Choking agents	54	135
Incapacitating agents	58	136
Incendiaries	60	138
Nerve agents	52*c–d*	129
Screening smokes	59	137
Tear agents	56	136
Vomiting agents	57	136
Transportation of sick and injured	46–48	103
Trench foot	41*a*	98
Two-man carry	48*k–o*	119
Unconsciousness	45	102
Veins	4*a*(2)(*b*)	5
Vital processes for life	4–5	4
Wounds:		
All	10–12, 15	24, 33
Minor	33	92
Severe:		
Abdominal	24	70
Chest, sucking	23	68
Face	22	68
Head	21	67
Neck	22	68

By Order of the Secretary of the Army:

W. C. WESTMORELAND,
General, United States Army,
Chief of Staff.

Official:

KENNETH G. WICKHAM
Major General, United States Army,
The Adjutant General.

Distribution:

Active Army, ARNG, USAR: To be distributed in accordance with DA Form 12–11 requirements for the Individual Soldier.

☆U.S. GOVERNMENT PRINTING OFFICE: 1974 540-823/7514B · 1-3